Temple Reset

Breaking Emotional Eating Patterns and
Rebuilding Sustainable Health

by

Joni Wilkinson

Copyright © 2026 by Joni Wilkinson.

All rights reserved.

No part of this book may be reproduced without written permission, except as permitted by U.S. copyright law. This publication is provided for informational purposes only and does not constitute legal, financial, or professional advice. The author and publisher make no warranties regarding accuracy or completeness and disclaim liability for any damages arising from its use. Readers should consult a qualified professional as needed. Web links may change over time. Opinions expressed are solely those of the author.

Scripture quotations are taken from the Holy Bible: New International Version® (NIV®), English Standard Version® (ESV®), and New Living Translation (NLT), used by permission. All rights reserved by their respective publishers.

Paperback ISBN: 979-8-9989413-0-6

Endorsements

This book is a powerful invitation to turn inward, offering gentle wisdom and practical tools for healing from the inside out. It reminds us that true transformation begins within, and that by tending to our inner world, we can reshape our outer reality. A must-read for anyone seeking wholeness, peace, and authentic self-discover.

- *Stacy Hardwick, MA, Licensed Professional Counselor specializing in Women Empowerment*

***

Joni Wilkinson has written a must-read spiritual guide for anyone struggling on their health and wellness journey.

-*Kristi Ross, Revitalized Wellness PLLC*

***

As a Licensed massage therapist, I have seen how deeply the body, mind, and spirit are connected. TEMPLE RESET offers a powerful and holistic approach to healing by encouraging a shift in your relationship with food while fostering spiritual and emotional well-being. This devotional not only guides you to nourish your body but also invites deeper reflection and connection with God. By combining daily scripture, prayer, and journaling, it empowers you to honor your body as a temple and embrace health, self-control, and balance. TEMPLE RESET is a transformative tool for anyone seeking a more intentional, holistic path to well-being.

-*Liz Creps, LMT*

I absolutely love how Joni gently leads our emotional needs back to God. Every void-filler, every cluttered corner of our hearts, minds, and bodies, she reminds us that sorting it all starts with Him. The wisdom she shares isn't just inspiring; it's a divine blueprint we can walk out daily. Partnering with the Holy Spirit is not optional; it's essential. I'm so proud of Joni and the healing work she's poured into this book. It's powerful; it's timely; and it's anointed.

-Kristal Klear, Founder OF ROCK PAPER SCISSORS FOUNDATION

***

Joni Wilkinson is deeply devoted to living a holistic life: spiritually, mentally, and emotionally. With unwavering authenticity and purpose, she pursues her God-given passions, remaining true to herself and refusing to let others sway her path. A powerful advocate, she stands boldly for those in danger, offering a voice and support to those seeking safety.

-Julie Nowacki, State Director of She Leads Oregon

***

In a world that glorifies hustle and quick fixes, Joni's devotional offers a sacred pause; an invitation to rediscover God's heart for nourishment, rest, and healing. Through Scripture, reflection, and a Christ-centered approach to food, this book gently guides readers toward a deeper relationship with the Lord, transforming not just the body, but the heart and spirit. It is a beautiful reminder that true restoration begins at His table.

-Jihya Harris, RN & Founder of Salt + Light Ministry

I have only known Joni for a couple of years, but in that short time, she has taught me so much about prayer and speaking God's promises over my life. I thought I had a personal relationship with Jesus before I met Joni, but learning how to pray has exponentially increased the joy in my everyday life and has given me new hope for my future.

-*Kimberly Caldwell MA Ed., Education Consultant*

Dedication

To my daughter, who has stood by my side through countless challenges, your love and support have been a constant source of strength. I am beyond grateful for you and the incredible woman you are becoming.

To my son, who has been a reminder of God's grace and purpose in my life: may you always walk in His light, knowing the value of discipline, health, and honoring your body as a temple.

To every woman who has felt broken, lost, or consumed by life's struggles, this book is for you. May you find healing, strength, and the courage to reset and align your body, mind, and spirit with God's perfect plan.

And to my Heavenly Father, for always being my refuge, my strength, and the One who has never left me, even in my darkest moments.

> *"It gave me great joy when some believers came and testified about your faithfulness to the truth, telling how you continue to walk in it."*
>
> 3 John 1:3 NIV.

Acknowledgement

To my children, your love and strength inspire me every day. Thank you for standing by me through it all.

To those who have shared their stories with me, your courage fuels this work. May it bring healing and hope to all who read it.

And to my Heavenly Father, thank You for guiding me, protecting me, and giving me the strength to share Your truth.

An Open Letter to the Reader

A Deeper Journey

Welcome to Temple Reset. This guide was prayerfully created for those who are ready to reset their body, mind, and spirit in alignment with God's purpose and presence. Over the next 21 days, you'll be invited into a deeper journey of healing, discipline, and renewal through scripture reflection, prayer, and journaling. Whether you feel stuck, weary, distracted, or hungry for more of God, this book is a space for you to quiet the noise, reset your focus, and reconnect with the truth of who you are in Christ.

My own journey into this reset wasn't just physical; it was spiritual and emotional. I found myself caught in unhealthy cycles: craving sweets, using food to numb pain, and obsessing over workouts. The more I tried to fix it, the worse I felt. I was worshiping comfort instead of the Comforter. Food had become an idol, and gluttony had taken root in a way I didn't recognize at first. But God, in His mercy, began to reveal that this wasn't about a diet; it was about surrender. He reminded me that my body is a temple of the Holy Spirit, and caring for it is an act of worship and obedience. As I laid down control, He began to restore not just my body, but my mind and spirit.

Inside Temple Reset, we'll explore key themes such as discipline (and how it's not punishment), gluttony and food idolatry, self-sabotage, spiritual clarity, and the lasting effects of childhood trauma on our health and choices. You'll find room to reflect, pray, and journal, real tools for a real reset.

This isn't just a book; it's an invitation to come back to the One who made you, to care for your temple with intentionality, and to walk in freedom. You don't have to stay stuck. God is a restorer, and He's ready to reset every part of you.

Thank you,

Joni Wilkinson

Preface

How to Apply Temple Reset to Your Life

Reset isn't just about changing how you eat; it's about healing your heart, mind, and spirit. Throughout this devotional, I want to challenge you to keep inviting God into your relationship with food and trust that He is leading you toward freedom, self-control, and health.

He has designed you with the ability to reset your relationship with food, shifting from obsession, emotional dependence, and unhealthy patterns to seeing food as fuel, a gift, and a tool for honoring God. Each day includes a scripture, reflection, prayer, and journaling prompt to guide your spiritual and physical transformation.

1 Corinthians 6:19–20 says, *"Do you not know that your bodies are temples of the Holy Spirit, who is in you, whom you have received from God? You are not your own; you were bought at a price. Therefore honor God with your bodies."*

Here are the key areas we will be unpacking:

1. Spiritual Reset

- Returning to your first love: Renewing your relationship with God.

- Letting go of distractions: Cutting out anything pulling you away from Him.
- Deepening your faith: Spending time in prayer, fasting, and reading His Word.

2. Emotional Reset

- Healing from past wounds: Allow God to deal with pain, trauma, or unforgiveness.
- Releasing burdens: Giving your worries, fears, and stresses to Him.
- Surrounding yourself with the right people: Being intentional about relationships that bring life, not drain it.

3. Physical Reset

- Taking care of your body: Rest, good nutrition, and exercise.
- Slowing down: Not running on empty but prioritizing balance.
- Honoring God with your health: Recognizing that your body is a temple and treating it as such.

In addition, you will begin to view your:

1. Your Body as God's Temple: Understanding how honoring your body through health and wellness is an act of worship.
2. Spiritual & Physical Renewal: Aligning weight loss goals with faith-based principles, focusing on transformation from the inside out.
3. Faith Over Frustration: Overcoming emotional and spiritual battles tied to weight and self-worth through biblical encouragement.

4. Discipline & Surrender: Learning the balance between discipline in health habits and surrendering control to God.
5. Biblical Nutrition & Stewardship: Exploring how scripture encourages wise choices in what we consume and how we care for our bodies.
6. Mindset & Motivation: Using scripture and prayer to combat doubt, fear, and discouragement.
7. Daily Devotions: Scripture-based reflections to keep faith at the center of the journey.
8. Prayer & Journaling Prompts: Encouraging self-reflection and connection with God throughout the process.

Each day of your journey, you will read a short devotion rooted in scripture. These reflections will encourage you to keep your focus on God as you go through the physical, mental, and emotional shifts of weight loss.

Let's Pray: "Lord, help me to see food as fuel and not as a source of comfort. Let me hunger for Your Word more than anything else. Strengthen me when I feel weak, and remind me that Your grace is sufficient in my struggles. Amen."

Prompt: What is one area where I have relied on food instead of God? How can I surrender that to Him today?

My Testimony: "I used to turn to food for comfort, but through this journey, I learned to turn to God instead. The weight loss was a blessing, but the real transformation happened inside AND outside."

Introduction

Sick and Tired of Being Sick and Tired

Easily food, and even fitness, can become idols when God isn't at the center. I was using food to soothe the pain of sadness, loneliness, and the weight of my divorce, thinking that working out would balance it out. But instead of true healing, it became another cycle, one idol replacing another.

We can deceive ourselves into thinking we are in control when, in reality, we're just shifting our dependence from one thing to another. Food was my comfort, but then exercise became my way of making up for it. Neither fully satisfied the deep ache in my soul. God was never in the midst because, at that time, my focus was on managing pain through physical means rather than spiritual surrender.

The more I tried to control things, the more out of control they became. Striving to fix ourselves through our own efforts can lead to even more frustration and isolation. I was doing everything "right" by society's standards: working out, trying to manage food, but without God at the center, the cycle just kept going.

No matter how many diets, workout plans, or videos I tried, they couldn't bring the healing or fulfillment I was searching for because God wasn't at the center. Without Him, we can strive and struggle, but we're left with the same emptiness. It's like trying to fix a broken chair with all the wrong tools; no matter how much effort you put in, it's not going to hold until you get to the root of the problem.

The missing piece was inviting God into that space, the part of my life where I felt lost, lonely, and disconnected. Once I acknowledged Him and allowed Him to reset my mindset, heart, and relationship with food and fitness, everything began to shift.

The shift in perspective, from self-reliance to God-reliance, only happen when God is the foundation; true transformation happen.

I had to learn my worth isn't based on what my body looks like or the number on the scale. It was a turning point where I started to understand that I am valuable because of God's love for me, not because of how I measure up to worldly standards. God has designed us to be healthy, not for superficial reasons, but so we can fulfill our purpose and live out His calling in our lives. Being healthy means honoring the body He's given us, nurturing it to have the strength and energy to do His work.

When we focus on our true worth in Him, it shifts our perspective. We stop chasing unattainable ideals and instead embrace the uniqueness of how He created us, flaws and all. Living in that freedom allows us to be fully present in our purpose, whether that's serving others, sharing His word, or doing what we were specifically designed for. It's not about perfection or comparison; it's about stewarding our bodies in a way that honors Him and equips us for the work He has for us here on earth.

Before My Own Temple Reset:

- Migraines, depression, anxiety; I was similarly taking the same medications that the celebrity Anna Nicole Smith was taking. "No, I can't die like this," I thought to myself. I made an internal decision for my life not to lead in the same direction. I was praying that I would become untied and untangled. I wasn't living right in my relationships; relationships with food and people were out of order, not in alignment. God was trying to get my attention, but since I did not do anything God's way, God was allowing me to get to the end of myself.

After:

- One's Purpose (my organization) was birthed during this time of prayer, fasting, and intentionally caring for my wellness.

Childhood Trauma

An Overlooked Food Disruptor

Childhood trauma and abuse can have a profound impact on weight gain due to factors like stress, emotional eating, hormonal imbalances, and the body's survival mechanisms. Trauma can trigger the release of cortisol, leading to increased fat storage, especially around the midsection. It can also create patterns of using food as comfort or a means of control.

When a child experiences trauma, whether physical, emotional, or sexual abuse, neglect, or even growing up in an unstable environment, their nervous system often shifts into a state of chronic stress. This activates the fight-or-flight response, which, when prolonged, can result in cortisol dysregulation, insulin resistance, and metabolic slowdown. The body learns to store fat as a protective measure, preparing for future stress or deprivation.

Additionally, trauma can disrupt the body's hunger and fullness cues. Many survivors turn to food for comfort, using it as a coping mechanism to numb pain, suppress emotions, or fill a void left by unmet needs in childhood. This can lead to emotional eating, binge eating, or even cycles of restriction and overconsumption. Some may develop an unhealthy relationship with food, associating it with safety or punishment.

Beyond the physical effects, childhood trauma often leads to low self-worth and a disconnect from the body. Many trauma survivors struggle with shame, feeling unworthy of care or health. They may not prioritize nutrition or exercise because, deep down, they don't believe they deserve to feel good. Others may subconsciously hold on to excess weight as a form of protection, believing that being smaller or more vulnerable could invite further harm.

Without healing, these patterns often follow individuals into adulthood, making weight loss difficult, not because of a lack of willpower, but because the body is holding on to past wounds. Resetting requires not just a physical shift but a mental, emotional, and spiritual transformation to break free from the chains of trauma.

Different types of childhood trauma affect weight in distinct ways, shaping a person's relationship with food, metabolism, and body image. Here's a breakdown of how various forms of trauma contribute to weight gain and difficulty losing weight:

1. Physical Abuse–Protection Through Weight

   - Children who experience physical abuse often develop a heightened sense of fear and hypervigilance. The body remains in a constant state of fight-or-flight, increasing cortisol production and leading to fat storage, particularly around the abdomen. Some survivors may subconsciously hold on to weight as a protective barrier, believing that being bigger will make them less of a target. Others may turn to food for comfort, seeking a sense of control over their bodies in an environment where they feel powerless.

2. Sexual Abuse–Dissociation and Self-Protection
   - Survivors of childhood sexual abuse often experience dissociation from their bodies as a way to cope with trauma. This detachment can lead to emotional eating, binge eating, or even disordered eating behaviors. Many survivors struggle with body shame, sometimes gaining weight subconsciously to become "invisible" or less desirable, thinking it might prevent further abuse. Others may restrict food intake, leading to cycles of starvation and bingeing, which damage metabolism over time.

3. Emotional and Verbal Abuse–Shame and Self-Sabotage
   - When a child is constantly criticized, shamed, or made to feel unworthy, they may develop an internal dialogue of self-hatred. This often results in self-sabotaging behaviors, such as overeating, poor nutrition, and lack of self-care. Many survivors struggle with chronic low self-esteem, believing they are not worth the effort to be healthy. Emotional abuse can also trigger stress-related eating, where food becomes a way to suppress emotions rather than process them.

4. Neglect–Food Scarcity Mindset and Binge Eating
   - Children who grow up in environments where food was scarce or inconsistent may develop a deep-rooted fear of hunger. This often leads to binge eating and hoarding food later in life, even when food is readily available. The brain and body remember the times of deprivation, causing them to store excess fat in case of future "famine." Additionally,

a lack of proper nutrition in childhood can disrupt metabolism and hormonal balance, making weight regulation more difficult.

5. Unstable or Chaotic Home Life–Chronic Stress and Cortisol Imbalance

- Children raised in unpredictable environments, where there was constant stress, arguing, substance abuse, or frequent moves, often experience chronic low-grade anxiety. This keeps cortisol levels elevated, making it harder to lose weight and easier to store fat. Many people who grew up in chaos develop food as a source of stability, using eating as a means to self-soothe in the absence of emotional security.

Distorted View of Self

A Destructive Cycle

Body dysmorphia, or Body Dysmorphic Disorder (BDD), is a mental health condition where a person becomes excessively preoccupied with perceived flaws in their appearance, flaws that are often unnoticeable to others. This obsession can lead to severe emotional distress, anxiety, and compulsive behaviors like excessive mirror-checking, comparing oneself to others, or engaging in extreme measures to "fix" the perceived flaw.

For Temple Reset, this can tie into the idea that our bodies are not the enemy but the temple of the Holy Spirit. When body image becomes an obsession, it can take our focus away from God's design and purpose for us. Instead of seeing our bodies as vessels to serve and glorify Him, we can fall into a cycle of striving, dissatisfaction, and even self-hatred.

A reset in this area would mean surrendering false perceptions, healing from the lies we've believed about ourselves, and learning to see our bodies as God sees them: fearfully and wonderfully made. It's about shifting from control and obsession to trust and alignment with His purpose.

Body dysmorphia, or Body Dysmorphic Disorder (BDD), is a mental health condition where a person becomes excessively preoccupied with perceived flaws in their appearance, flaws that are often unnoticeable to others. This obsession can lead to severe emotional distress, anxiety, and compulsive behaviors like excessive mirror-checking, comparing oneself to others, or engaging in extreme measures to "fix" the perceived flaw. But body dysmorphia isn't just about appearance; it's often deeply rooted in trauma, shame, and a distorted sense of self.

For many, body dysmorphia doesn't appear out of nowhere; it can be the result of childhood wounds, abuse, rejection, or experiences that made them feel unworthy or not enough. Trauma, especially in the form of sexual abuse, domestic violence, or emotional neglect, can disconnect a person from their body, making them feel unsafe in their own skin. The body becomes a battlefield, something to control, shrink, hide, or punish, rather than a temple of the Holy Spirit.

This is crucial because it's not just about breaking free from obsessive thoughts about appearance; it's about healing the deeper wounds that led to them. When trauma is unresolved, it speaks lies over our identity. It tells us we are damaged, unlovable, or out of control. We then try to regain control through extreme dieting, excessive exercise, self-harm, or even avoiding mirrors entirely, only to find that no amount of external change fixes the internal pain.

A true reset means going beyond the surface. It means surrendering false perceptions, healing from the lies we've believed about ourselves, and learning to see our bodies as God sees them, fearfully and wonderfully made. It's about shifting from control and obsession to trust and alignment with His purpose. It means recognizing that our worth is not in how we look, but in who we are in Christ. And it means allowing God to restore what trauma stole, bringing wholeness to both body and soul.

Trauma distorts identity, warps perception, and often leaves people feeling disconnected from their own bodies, emotions, and even God. But restoration comes when we allow Him to reset our hearts, minds, and bodies back to His original design. Here's how:

Recognizing the Lies and Replacing Them with Truth

Trauma plants deep-seated lies: You are unworthy. You are broken. You are beyond healing. These lies shape how we see ourselves and our bodies. The first step toward restoration is identifying these lies and replacing them with God's truth. Romans 12:2 reminds us to be transformed by the renewing of our minds. This means actively speaking and meditating on what God says about us: You are fearfully and wonderfully made (Psalm 139:14). You are a new creation (2 Corinthians 5:17). You are deeply loved (Jeremiah 31:3).

Inviting God into the Pain

God doesn't heal what we hide. Restoration begins when we bring our wounds, memories, and brokenness before Him. This can happen through deep prayer, journaling, or even speaking aloud to Him about the things that hurt the most. Psalm 34:18 says that the Lord is near to the brokenhearted and saves the crushed in spirit. He wants to step into the very places where trauma stole joy, peace, and identity.

Releasing Control and Surrendering the Body

For many, trauma leads to a desperate need to control, whether through food, exercise, appearance, or self-protection. But true healing requires surrender. We must release the body back to its original purpose: a temple of the Holy Spirit (1 Corinthians 6:19-20), not an object to perfect, punish, or fear. This surrender isn't about neglecting health, but about resetting our perspective to care for our bodies in a way that honors God rather than fuels anxiety, comparison, or shame.

Forgiveness as a Pathway to Freedom

Unforgiveness chains us to the very trauma that wounded us. This doesn't mean excusing what happened, but it does mean releasing those who hurt us into God's hands. Matthew 6:14-15 reminds us that forgiveness is essential, not just for others, but for our own healing. When we forgive, we break the cycle of trauma's grip and allow God to restore peace in our hearts.

Reclaiming What Was Stolen

Trauma often steals joy, confidence, relationships, and a sense of safety. But restoration means stepping back into those things with boldness. Maybe it's allowing yourself to laugh again, to wear clothes you once avoided, to move your body in ways that bring joy instead of punishment, or to trust people again. Joel 2:25 declares that God will restore the years the locusts have eaten; He is a God of redemption.

Living in Identity, Not in Wounds

At the core of restoration is the realization that we are not what happened to us; we are who God says we are. Trauma may be part of our story, but it does not define our identity. God restores by giving beauty for ashes (Isaiah 61:3) and turning pain into purpose. When we walk in the fullness of who He created us to be, we reclaim every part of ourselves that trauma tried to erase.

Our Food Relationship

Learning the Ways of Nourishment

Having a good relationship with food means viewing food as nourishment rather than as something to control, fear, or use as an emotional crutch. It involves listening to your body's natural hunger and fullness cues, enjoying a variety of foods without guilt, and understanding that food is meant to fuel your body, not define your worth.

A healthy relationship with food includes:

- Balance: Eating a variety of foods, including both nutritious and enjoyable treats, without extreme restrictions.
- Freedom from Guilt: Not labeling foods as "good" or "bad" but understanding that all foods can fit in moderation.
- Mindful Eating: Being present while eating, savoring flavors, and recognizing when you're truly hungry or full.
- No Emotional Dependence: Not using food as a primary way to cope with emotions like stress, loneliness, or boredom.
- Trusting Your Body: Eating when you're hungry, stopping when you're satisfied, and recognizing that your body knows what it needs.

Having a good relationship with food means aligning how we nourish our bodies with God's design and purpose. Our bodies are temples of the Holy Spirit, and food should serve as fuel to sustain, restore, and energize us, not as an idol or an enemy.

A Temple Reset Approach to Food:

- Stewardship, Not Control: Instead of obsessing over food, we recognize it as a gift from God, using it wisely without allowing it to master us.
- Freedom Over Shame: No food is inherently sinful, and eating should not be tied to guilt or legalism. It's about balance and wisdom, not restriction and punishment.
- Nourishment, Not Numbing: Food should fuel our bodies for God's work, not be a way to suppress emotions, loneliness, or spiritual emptiness.
- Listening to the Spirit & the Body: Just as we seek God's voice in our spiritual walk, we can tune in to how He designed our bodies, eating when hungry, stopping when satisfied, and choosing foods that bring strength and vitality.
- Joy and Gratitude: Enjoying food in a way that brings gratitude to God, recognizing that He provides not just for survival but for delight and fellowship.

Resetting our relationship with food means surrendering it to God, breaking cycles of obsession or avoidance, and choosing to honor Him with how we fuel our bodies.

Accepted Addictions

Hijacking the Brain, Enslaving the Body

No one is better than anyone else; we all have struggles, strongholds, and things we turn to instead of God. Addiction, whether to drugs, food, sugar, work, or anything else, is often a symptom of a deeper issue, like pain, trauma, or unmet needs.

Jesus made it clear that self-righteousness is a dangerous trap. In Luke 18:9-14, He told the parable of the Pharisee and the tax collector; one thought he was better because of his outward righteousness, while the other humbly admitted his need for mercy. The tax collector, who acknowledged his sin, was the one justified before God.

Unfortunately, some Christians can fall into the same trap as the Pharisee, judging others while ignoring their own struggles. But true Christianity is about humility, grace, and recognizing that we all need Jesus. Whether someone is addicted to heroin or sugar, both reveal a dependency on something other than God for comfort, escape, or fulfillment.

Addiction is often misunderstood because people tend to categorize it; some addictions, like drugs or alcohol, are seen as more destructive, while socially accepted ones, like sugar, food, or even workaholism, are often ignored. But in reality, addiction in any form hijacks the brain, enslaves the body, and keeps people from living in true freedom.

Here are some keys for Temple Reset on Addiction:

1. Addiction Isn't Just About Drugs & Alcohol
   - The brain reacts to sugar, carbs, and processed foods similarly to how it reacts to drugs. Dopamine spikes create cravings and withdrawal symptoms.
   - Emotional eating, binge eating, and food obsession can be just as controlling as substance addiction.
   - Other addictions include social media, validation, pornography, work, shopping, caffeine, and even toxic relationships.

2. Spiritual and Physical Bondage
   - Addiction of any kind keeps people from being fully surrendered to God.
   - The enemy loves to keep people trapped in cycles of dependency, whether it's on substances, food, or destructive habits.
   - Breaking addiction is about more than willpower; it requires healing at the root, physically, mentally, and spiritually.

3. The Hidden Dangers of Sugar, Carbs & Processed Foods
   - Studies show sugar is more addictive than cocaine in some cases.
   - Processed foods are designed to create cravings and overconsumption.
   - Food addiction leads to inflammation, disease, and mental health struggles like depression and anxiety.

4. The Church & Hypocrisy Around Addiction
   - Many Christians condemn drug addicts while being addicted to food, caffeine, or social media.
   - Gluttony is rarely preached about, but it's just as destructive.
   - True freedom comes from surrendering all addictions, not just the ones society looks down on.
5. Breaking Free & Resetting the Temple
   - Fasting and detoxing can help reset the body and break food addictions.
   - Renewing the mind through Scripture and prayer is key to overcoming addiction.
   - True healing means replacing addiction with God's presence, not just swapping one dependency for another.

The root of gluttony often goes deeper than just the physical act of overeating. It can be tied to emotional emptiness or unresolved trauma. Many turn to food as a coping mechanism, using it to fill a void created by feelings of sadness, anxiety, or past wounds. This creates an unhealthy relationship with food, where eating becomes a way to soothe emotional pain instead of nourishing the body.

At times, gluttony stems from a lack of self-control or discipline. An inability to regulate desires and impulses, especially when it comes to food, can reveal an underlying issue of self-mastery. For some, food offers a temporary distraction from stress, discomfort, or personal struggles. The momentary pleasure it provides becomes an escape, preventing the individual from facing deeper emotional or spiritual concerns.

Cultural or societal influences can also play a significant role in the development of gluttony. Food often becomes intertwined with socialization, celebration, and status. People may overeat to fit in or because food is abundant and often seen as a source of comfort or joy in gatherings.

Ultimately, gluttony may point to a deeper spiritual void. When people feel disconnected or unfulfilled in their relationship with God, they may turn to food for satisfaction, looking for something to fill the emptiness that only a close connection with Him can truly heal. Healing from gluttony requires addressing these deeper emotional and spiritual root causes, realigning with God's purpose, and finding true fulfillment in His presence.

Overeating

An Emotional Crutch

Overeating is more than just consuming too much food; it's often a symptom of something deeper. It's when food becomes an emotional crutch or a way to avoid confronting life's challenges. While eating is a basic and essential act for survival, overeating occurs when it goes beyond our body's needs, often driven by emotional triggers like stress, sadness, or even boredom. In these moments, we may seek comfort in food, attempting to fill a void or numb uncomfortable feelings.

The harm of overeating goes far beyond the immediate discomfort of being full. Physically, it can put undue stress on the body, leading to weight gain, obesity, and other serious health issues such as diabetes, heart disease, and digestive problems. These physical issues can, in turn, create emotional burdens, guilt, shame, and frustration that feed into the cycle of overeating.

Spiritually, overeating can create a disconnect between the body, mind, and spirit. It's a form of self-neglect that undermines the health and vitality God designed us to have. When food is used to fulfill emotional or spiritual needs that only God can satisfy, we miss out on the nourishment of His presence, which is the true source of our peace and fulfillment.

Overeating also takes away from our ability to live in balance and moderation, which are key aspects of honoring the body as a temple. It keeps us stuck in a cycle of unhealthy dependence on food, rather than learning to rely on God's strength to meet our true needs. To reset and reclaim health, it's essential to examine the reasons behind overeating, address the underlying emotional or spiritual causes, and realign our choices with the purpose and intention that God has for our bodies.

Did you grow up in a household where you were expected or even rewarded for "cleaning your plate" at dinnertime? For many of us, this phrase was a common refrain during childhood, an expectation rooted in the belief that finishing all the food on your plate was a sign of discipline and gratitude. While well-intentioned, this practice can inadvertently plant the seeds of unhealthy relationships with food that persist into adulthood.

In a household where cleaning your plate was strongly emphasized, you may have been conditioned to ignore your body's natural signals of fullness. Instead of learning to listen to your internal cues, whether you're satisfied, content, or truly hungry, the focus was on finishing everything in front of you, regardless of your body's needs. This conditioning can create a mindset that food must always be consumed in its entirety and that leaving food behind is wasteful or unacceptable, even when you're no longer hungry.

This way of thinking can lead to overeating and an unhealthy attachment to food. It makes it harder to trust your body's wisdom, as the practice of "cleaning your plate" overrides the signals that help you distinguish between when you're actually full and when you're simply eating because it's expected. Over time, this mindset can foster guilt or anxiety around food, especially if you've been taught that food is scarce or that not finishing your meal means you're ungrateful.

In the context of "Temple Reset," this practice challenges us to rethink the relationship between our bodies and food. God has designed us to be mindful stewards of our bodies, and part of that stewardship is recognizing when we've had enough to eat. The key is finding balance, honoring our body's natural hunger and fullness cues, embracing moderation, and breaking free from habits or expectations that may not serve our physical, emotional, or spiritual well-being.

Did you feel, either as a child or even now, that food was scarce in your household? Was your family large, and if you didn't get yours, it might not be there later? For some, these experiences were a significant part of growing up, and they can leave lasting emotional impressions on how we view food as adults.

In a household where food is scarce, or where there's an unspoken competition for it, the anxiety of not getting enough can shape how we approach meals. As a child, if you were in a large family where food was limited, it could create a sense of urgency to grab as much as you could, as fast as you could, because there was a fear that if you didn't, you might go without. This can lead to eating quickly, not paying attention to fullness, and overeating out of a sense of scarcity or insecurity. The experience of watching food disappear fast, or seeing others compete for portions, can create a belief that food is something to hoard rather than something to be enjoyed in moderation.

This mindset doesn't just stop at childhood. Even into adulthood, the emotional scars of this fear of scarcity can influence how we approach food. People who grew up in this kind of environment may find it difficult to leave food behind on their plates, even when they're full. They may eat in excess to ensure they don't go hungry, as if the experience of scarcity as a child still looms over them.

In the context of "Temple Reset," it's important to address this emotional relationship with food. Scarcity and fear may have once been real experiences, but they do not need to define how we nourish our bodies today. God's provision is abundant, and while there are seasons of challenge and need, there is also a call to trust Him and His promises. The idea of "taking only what we need" reflects this shift from scarcity to abundance. It's about trusting that the Lord will provide, not just in physical nourishment, but in emotional and spiritual fullness as well. Healing and resetting the relationship with food often require letting go of old patterns tied to past fears, learning to embrace moderation, and trusting that we don't have to overindulge to ensure we're cared for.

Perhaps, as a child, you were given ice cream or some other dessert after you'd eaten all your dinner. Even if you weren't hungry, you may have eaten the dessert because it was presented as a reward. "Clean your plate, and you'll get something sweet!" was a phrase many of us grew up hearing. While this may have seemed harmless or even joyful in the moment, it's an example of learned behaviors that can shape our relationship with food in ways we don't always recognize.

This pattern of using food as a reward teaches us that eating is not only about nourishment but also about seeking external rewards or validation. Food, especially sweet or indulgent foods, becomes associated with comfort, pleasure, and sometimes even achievement. Over time, this connection creates a desire to seek out food, not for nourishment, but for the emotional satisfaction or reward it promises. This can lead to overeating, especially when we're not truly hungry, simply because we've learned that food provides a sense of reward, relief, or pleasure.

As we grow older, this learned behavior can be difficult to break. We may find ourselves reaching for sweets or indulgent foods in moments of stress, boredom, or celebration, even when we're not physically hungry. The habit of eating as a way to feel good or receive some form of reward can become ingrained, influencing our choices in ways that don't necessarily align with our body's needs or our overall health.

In the context of "Temple Reset," this kind of learned behavior challenges us to shift our perspective on food. Instead of associating food with rewards or emotional coping, we need to reconnect with the purpose of nourishment and the true source of satisfaction, which comes from God. Recognizing that our bodies are temples and deserve to be treated with honor and respect means understanding that food should fuel us, not just emotionally or mentally but also physically. Resetting this mindset involves breaking free from using food as a reward and learning to listen to our bodies' true needs. It's about finding fulfillment not in the temporary pleasure of food but in the deeper satisfaction that comes from living in alignment with God's purpose for our lives and bodies.

Our bodies are designed to use food as fuel, and just like any machine, they have a certain capacity for how much fuel they can handle. The stomach, although it can stretch to accommodate larger amounts of food, is a relatively small organ, about the size of a person's fist when it's empty. It's made up of muscles that allow it to expand and contract, helping us digest and process the food we consume. But what happens when we continually overeat, beyond our body's natural capacity?

When we binge eat regularly, the stomach is constantly stretched far beyond its normal size. Although it can stretch to accommodate large amounts of food, it isn't meant to be in a stretched state all the time. This repeated overstretching doesn't give the stomach the opportunity to return to its natural, more compact shape. Over time, the muscles of the stomach may adapt to this constant expansion, and it may start to require more food to feel full. This can lead to a vicious cycle of overeating, as the stomach's "normal" size becomes larger and larger, which in turn leads to greater quantities of food being consumed.

Continual overeating and the chronic stretching of the stomach can have significant health impacts. For one, it can strain the digestive system and lead to discomfort, bloating, and other gastrointestinal issues. The constant need for more food can also create a dependency on larger portions to feel satisfied, which may lead to weight gain and associated health problems like obesity, diabetes, and heart disease. Additionally, consistently overeating can dull the body's natural hunger cues, making it harder to distinguish between real hunger and emotional or habitual eating.

From a spiritual perspective, this cycle of overeating can be seen as a disconnection between the body and its natural, God-designed limits. Our bodies were created with a need for balance and moderation. Yet, when we overeat regularly, we disregard the signals that God gave us to guide us to healthy living. Resetting this pattern involves not only taking physical steps to restore balance to the body but also addressing the emotional or spiritual reasons we may turn to food for comfort or satisfaction.

By learning to respect the body's natural limits, we can foster a healthier, more balanced relationship with food. This means giving our stomachs a chance to return to their normal size, learning to listen to our body's hunger cues, and understanding that we don't need to overindulge to feel fulfilled. Instead, we can find true satisfaction in moderation and in honoring the body as a temple, which is what God intended for us.

Food Idolatry

From Comfort to Nourishment

Food idolatry is when food takes a place in our lives that it was never meant to have, when it becomes a source of comfort, identity, or control instead of being seen as a provision from God. It can show up in different ways, such as emotional eating, obsession with diets, or placing too much emphasis on certain foods for fulfillment rather than looking to God for satisfaction.

Food idolatry could be explored in the context of how we allow food to dictate our emotions, self-worth, and even our spiritual well-being. Scripture reminds us that our bodies are temples of the Holy Spirit (1 Corinthians 6:19-20), meaning we should be mindful of what we consume, not just physically, but spiritually and emotionally as well.

This doesn't mean food is bad or that enjoying it is wrong. God created food to nourish and sustain us, and even to bring joy and community. But when food becomes an escape, a coping mechanism, or an idol that takes the place of God, it can hinder our spiritual and physical health. Resetting the temple means realigning our relationship with food to reflect God's design, using it as fuel, enjoying it in moderation, and ultimately finding our fulfillment in Him, not in what's on our plate.

Using food as comfort is one of the most common ways food becomes an idol in our lives. It happens when we turn to food to soothe our emotions, whether it's stress, sadness, boredom, loneliness, or even celebration, rather than turning to God. This pattern often starts subtly but can become a deeply ingrained habit, shaping our relationship with both food and our faith.

Gluttony

The Enemy's Plan of Distortion

Gluttony is one of the ways the enemy distorts our relationship with food. The Bible warns against it in Proverbs 23:20-21, saying, *"Do not join those who drink too much wine or gorge themselves on meat, for drunkards and gluttons become poor, and drowsiness clothes them in rags."* Gluttony is not just about overeating; it is about allowing food to control you rather than submitting your body to the Lord's will. It creates a cycle of indulgence and guilt, leaving you feeling physically sluggish and spiritually empty.

Philippians 3:19 speaks of those whose "god is their stomach." When we turn to food for comfort, stress relief, or emotional fulfillment instead of turning to God, we are making an idol out of it. This doesn't mean food is bad; God created food for our nourishment and enjoyment, but it is not meant to be our source of peace, joy, or identity.

Self-control is a fruit of the Spirit, and God calls us to exercise it in every area of our lives, including how we eat. Galatians 5:22-23 reminds us that when we walk in the Spirit, we develop self-control. This doesn't mean restriction or legalism; it means honoring our bodies by listening to them and seeking God's guidance in our choices. Food should be enjoyed with gratitude, not worshiped or misused.

At its core, gluttony and food obsession are symptoms of a deeper issue: an unfulfilled hunger for God. Matthew 4:4 says, *"Man shall not live on bread alone, but on every word that comes from the mouth of God."* True satisfaction does not come from overeating, restricting, or controlling food; it comes from being filled with God's presence.

Breaking free from the grip of food fixation starts with surrender. If you've struggled with gluttony, food addiction, or an unhealthy relationship with eating, know that God's grace is bigger. 1 Corinthians 10:13 reminds us that He always provides a way out of temptation. Bring this area before Him, asking for wisdom, self-control, and a renewed perspective on food.

A prayer for release: Lord, I repent for the times I have allowed food to become an idol in my life. I surrender my cravings, my struggles, and my relationship with eating to You. Teach me self-control and help me to see food as a good gift, not a master. Satisfy me with Your presence and help me to live in freedom. In Jesus' name, Amen.

God does not call us to a life of bondage, to food, to guilt, or to worldly expectations. He calls us to freedom. When we reset our perspective on food, we step into the abundant life He designed for us.

The Root of Comfort Eating

Seeking True Satisfaction

Food is one of the earliest comforts we experience; babies cry, and they are fed. There's nothing wrong with enjoying food or associating it with warmth and connection, but when it becomes our primary means of coping, it can create a cycle of dependence. Instead of bringing our burdens to God, we may reach for food to fill an emotional void, numb pain, or create a temporary sense of relief.

Food and the Flesh vs. the Spirit

The Bible warns about living according to the desires of the flesh rather than the Spirit (Galatians 5:16-17). Comfort eating often feeds the flesh, offering a quick fix but leaving the deeper issue unresolved. This can lead to guilt, shame, and an even greater reliance on food as a crutch. Jesus invites us to come to Him when we are weary and burdened (Matthew 11:28), but food often becomes the more immediate, tangible source of comfort, one that never truly satisfies.

The Illusion of Control

Food as comfort can also be linked to control. When life feels chaotic, food can feel like one thing we can regulate. Some turn to overeating, while others restrict or obsess over what they eat. In both cases, food becomes a misplaced source of security. The enemy uses this as a distraction, keeping us preoccupied with our physical cravings instead of seeking the deep peace that only comes from God.

Resetting the Temple: A Biblical Perspective

1. Recognizing the Pattern: The first step in breaking food idolatry is identifying when and why we seek comfort in food. Are we eating because we're physically hungry, or are we feeding an emotional hunger?
2. Replacing the Craving with God's Presence: Psalm 34:8 says, "Taste and see that the Lord is good." Instead of turning to food in moments of stress or sadness, we can turn to prayer, worship, or Scripture, allowing God to be our source of peace.
3. Honoring the Body as a Temple: When we see our bodies as vessels of the Holy Spirit, it shifts our perspective. Rather than indulging in food for escape, we choose nourishment that fuels our purpose and well-being.
4. Finding Comfort in Community: Many times, food is used to fill a relational void. Instead of eating in isolation, we can seek connection with a godly community, where we can process emotions in a healthy way.

Breaking Free from Food as Comfort

Resetting our relationship with food doesn't mean we can't enjoy it, it means we enjoy it in the way God intended: as fuel, as a gift, and as part of fellowship. True comfort comes from the Holy Spirit, not from a full stomach. When we shift our dependence from food to God, we experience the deeper satisfaction that no meal can provide.

Hyper-Focus & Food

When Control Becomes Captivity

Hyper-focus can be a powerful tool, allowing us to accomplish great things. But when it comes to food, it can turn into an exhausting and deceptive form of bondage. It often starts with good intentions, being mindful of what we eat, taking care of our bodies, and striving for health. But somewhere along the way, that focus can shift from discipline to obsession.

I didn't realize at first that I was caught in this cycle. What began as a desire to be healthier became an all-consuming fixation. Food was no longer just fuel; it was a constant calculation. I tracked everything: what to eat, when to eat, and how much to eat. I researched every nutrient, every calorie, and every possible way to optimize my body. I thought I was in control, but the truth was, food was controlling me.

The more I hyper-focused, the more my body resisted. I wasn't thriving; I was trapped. Despite my best efforts, my body was getting bigger, my mind was exhausted, and my spirit was drained. I was doing everything "right," yet something felt deeply wrong.

Then God revealed the truth: my hyper-focus on food wasn't just about food. It was about control. It was about filling a void, trying to fix something deeper within me. Food had become an idol, something I was relying on more than I was relying on Him.

The Bible warns us about the danger of allowing anything other than God to have mastery over our lives:

"Everything is permissible for me," but not everything is beneficial. "Everything is permissible for me," but I will not be mastered by anything." — 1 Corinthians 6:12 (NIV)

I was allowing food to master me. I had convinced myself I was simply being diligent, but in reality, I was in bondage. I had taken something good: nutrition, health, discipline, and turned it into an idol. And just like every other idol, it over-promised and under-delivered. Instead of peace, I had anxiety. Instead of freedom, I felt trapped.

The moment of breakthrough came when I surrendered. I laid it all at the feet of Jesus. I stopped tracking, stopped obsessing, and stopped believing the lie that I had to control everything. Instead, I started listening to my body, to my spirit, and most importantly, to God.

The Lord reminded me of Matthew 6:25, where Jesus tells us:

"Therefore I tell you, do not worry about your life, what you will eat or drink; or about your body, what you will wear. Isn't life more than food, and the body more than clothes?"

God didn't create us to live in cycles of obsession, anxiety, and striving. He created us to live in freedom. But that freedom only comes when we trust Him more than we trust ourselves.

This is what Temple Reset is all about: not another diet, not another formula, but a true realignment of body, mind, and spirit with the way God designed us to live. It's about breaking free from anything that enslaves us, including the hyper-focus that keeps us trapped.

Food is a gift, but it is not a god. My body is a temple, but it is not my master. The only way to truly reset was to let God be God, to surrender control and let Him bring the healing, peace, and balance I so desperately needed.

"So if the Son sets you free, you will be free indeed." — John 8:36 (NIV)

I don't have to be ruled by food anymore. And neither do you.

Application–Take a moment to reflect:

- Are there areas of your life where focus has turned into fixation?
- Have you allowed food, fitness, or any other pursuit to take up more space in your heart than it should?
- What would it look like to surrender this area to God today?

True freedom comes when we release control and trust God with every part of our lives, including our bodies. John 8:36 reminds us, "So if the Son sets you free, you will be free indeed."

Prayer:

Lord, I surrender my need for control. I don't want to be mastered by anything other than You. Help me to reset my focus and trust You with my body, mind, and spirit. Show me how to live in the freedom You have called me to. In Jesus' name, Amen.

Challenge:

Today, choose one small way to surrender. Maybe it's skipping the food tracking, resting instead of over-exercising, or simply thanking God for your body instead of criticizing it. Let today be a step toward true freedom.

Reset Challenge:

Spend intentional time with God, laying down every burden, fear, or stronghold. Commit to walking in the freedom He offers.

This journey is about more than just food or fitness; it's about true transformation, aligning your temple with God's purpose.

Aligning your body with God's purpose means recognizing that it was created for His glory, not for the indulgence of fleshly desires. 1 Corinthians 6:19-20 reminds us that our bodies are temples of the Holy Spirit, and we are called to honor God with them. When food becomes an idol, something we obsess over, depend on for comfort, or use it to fill an emotional or spiritual void, it takes a place in our hearts that belongs to God alone.

The Root of Self-Sabotage

The Hidden Why

Self-sabotage is often rooted in deeper emotional, spiritual, and psychological struggles that keep us from fully stepping into the healing and wholeness God desires for us.

Why Do We Self-Sabotage?

Unresolved Trauma & Pain

When we've experienced hurt, rejection, or abuse, we may unconsciously believe we are unworthy of healing, success, or love. The pain becomes familiar, and stepping into something new, even something good, can feel unsafe.

Fear of Change or Responsibility

Healing and transformation require change, and change can be uncomfortable. Sometimes, we sabotage our progress because staying in dysfunction feels easier than facing the unknown. There's also a fear of the responsibility that comes with wholeness; when we're healed, we no longer have excuses to stay stuck.

Misperceptions of Identity

If we've been conditioned to believe we are broken, weak, or incapable, we'll continue to act in ways that reinforce that belief.

We may say we want freedom, but if deep down we believe we're unworthy of it, we will unconsciously sabotage our progress.

Cycles of Shame & Condemnation

The enemy loves to trap us in a cycle of shame, making us feel guilty for our struggles and then convincing us that because we've failed before, we'll fail again. This keeps us from moving forward and receiving the grace God freely offers.

Emotional Comfort in Destructive Patterns

Whether it's food, addiction, toxic relationships, or overworking, self-sabotage often comes from seeking comfort in things that ultimately harm us. These coping mechanisms provide temporary relief but pull us further from true healing.

Spiritual Warfare

There is a real enemy who does not want us to walk in freedom. If he can keep us trapped in patterns of self-sabotage, he can keep us from fulfilling the calling God has for us. Recognizing this battle is key to overcoming it.

Breaking the Cycle

Renewing the Mind: Aligning our thoughts with God's truth instead of lies from the past.

Healing the Heart: Allowing God to go to the root of our wounds instead of numbing them.

Resetting the Body: Honoring our physical temple with nourishment, movement, and rest in a way that aligns with God's design, not culture's expectations.

Walking in Authority: Recognizing that we are not victims; we have the power, through Christ, to break cycles and walk in victory.

Self-sabotage loses its grip when we address the deeper reasons behind it and invite God into every part of our healing. Temple Reset isn't just about resetting habits; it's about resetting the way we see ourselves through God's eyes and stepping fully into the freedom He has for us.

Self-Sabotage & Self-Worth

Breaking the Cycle

Self-sabotage is when we consciously or unconsciously undermine our own progress, success, or well-being. It's the behaviors, thoughts, or habits that keep us stuck, even when we desperately want change. It can manifest in many ways: procrastination, negative self-talk, destructive eating habits, avoidance, or even quitting just before a breakthrough. At its core, self-sabotage is often tied to our sense of self-worth.

Why Do We Self-Sabotage?

Self-sabotage is usually rooted in fear, past wounds, or deep-seated beliefs about who we are and what we deserve. Here are some key reasons why we do it:

1. Fear of Failure: If we fail, it confirms the lies we've believed about ourselves: that we're not good enough, smart enough, or strong enough. So instead, we sabotage before we even get the chance to succeed.
2. Fear of Success: Success can be uncomfortable if we don't feel worthy of it. Sometimes, we fear the responsibility, expectations, or changes that come with it.
3. Unresolved Trauma: Past hurts can keep us trapped in cycles of pain, making us believe we don't deserve healing, joy, or freedom.
4. Comfort in Familiarity: Even if something is destructive, if it's familiar, it feels "safe." We stay in patterns that we know, even when they harm us.

5. Spiritual Attack: The enemy comes to "steal, kill, and destroy," (John 10:10). If he can get us to sabotage ourselves, he doesn't even have to do the work.

Overcoming Self-Sabotage

Breaking free from self-sabotage starts with understanding who we are in Christ and replacing lies with truth.

1. Renew Your Mind: The Bible says to *"take every thought captive,"* (2 Corinthians 10:5). Recognize destructive thought patterns and replace them with God's truth.
2. Embrace Your Worth: Your worth is not in your past, your mistakes, or what others have spoken over you. You are a child of God, fearfully and wonderfully made (Psalm 139:14).
3. Practice Discipline as Worship: Discipline isn't punishment; it's a tool for freedom. When you deny the flesh, you strengthen the spirit (Galatians 5:16).
4. Take Small, Consistent Steps: Progress is built on daily choices. Don't wait for motivation, build habits that align with who God says you are.
5. Stay Accountable: Surround yourself with people who will call out the sabotage and remind you of your purpose.
6. Walk in Grace : If you mess up, don't let shame drag you back into old cycles. Repent, reset, and move forward.

God doesn't call us to live in defeat. He calls us to walk in freedom. The moment we start seeing ourselves through His eyes, self-sabotage loses its power. Every time you resist the urge to self-destruct, you're taking one more step toward the abundant life God has for you.

Boundaries

Guarding the Temple

Just as a physical temple has gates and walls to protect what is sacred inside, our lives require boundaries to safeguard our bodies, minds, and spirits. Boundaries are not restrictions meant to punish us; they are divine safeguards designed to keep us on the path God has called us to walk. Without them, we open ourselves to distractions, temptations, and destructive patterns that pull us away from His presence and purpose.

Many people struggle with boundaries because they associate them with limitation or legalism, but true boundaries, God-given boundaries, are about protection and alignment. They help us stay focused on what matters most and prevent unnecessary pain, confusion, and regret. If we don't establish and enforce boundaries in every area of our lives, we will end up drained, distracted, and vulnerable to attacks from the enemy.

Boundaries in the Body

In the same way that we are mindful of what enters a place of worship, we must be mindful of what we allow into our bodies. The foods we consume either fuel us for God's work or hinder our ability to function effectively. Our bodies were created to thrive, not merely survive, but what we put into them determines how well they function.

When we don't set boundaries with food, we can fall into cycles of indulgence, regret, and self-sabotage. I've been there, eating to numb emotions, reaching for sugar or junk food to cope with stress, then feeling even worse afterward. Without boundaries, our flesh takes over, dictating what we eat, how much we eat, and why we eat. But when we recognize that our bodies are temples of the Holy Spirit (1 Corinthians 6:19-20), we start treating them with honor.

Boundaries with food don't mean deprivation; they mean discipline. Learning to say no to what weakens us and yes to what strengthens us is an act of stewardship. It's about fueling our bodies with what helps us stay clear-minded, energetic, and strong enough to fulfill our purpose. It's about listening to the Holy Spirit rather than our cravings.

Just as food is fuel, sleep, movement, and rest also require boundaries. If we don't prioritize these, we will find ourselves burned out, sick, and ineffective. Our bodies need rest to reset, just as God commanded a Sabbath. If we ignore the need for balance, we become physically and spiritually depleted, unable to function at the level God desires for us.

Boundaries in the Mind

The Bible tells us to take every thought captive (2 Corinthians 10:5) because our thought life directs our actions. If we don't guard our minds, we will be consumed with lies, lies about our worth, our identity, and our ability to overcome. Setting mental boundaries means choosing what we dwell on, what voices we allow to speak into our lives, and what we meditate on daily.

We live in a world that constantly bombards us with distractions, negativity, and temptations. If we are not intentional about filtering what we allow into our minds, we will be shaped by the world rather than by the Word of God. Social media, entertainment, and even conversations we engage in can either uplift us or drain us. Setting mental boundaries means being mindful of what we expose ourselves to and how it affects our thoughts and emotions.

Mental boundaries also mean refusing to dwell on toxic thoughts, whether they are self-critical thoughts, fear-based thoughts, or the lies of the enemy. If we don't take control of our minds, our minds will control us. How many times have you let a single negative thought spiral into a full-blown attack on your confidence, peace, or joy? Thoughts have power, and without boundaries, they can lead us into discouragement, anxiety, and even self-destruction.

Instead of allowing harmful thoughts to run unchecked, we must replace them with truth. God's Word is the ultimate mental boundary; it separates truth from deception, faith from fear, and hope from despair. Renewing our minds daily in the Word of God transforms the way we think, respond, and live (Romans 12:2).

Boundaries in the Spirit

Spiritual boundaries ensure that we don't become lukewarm, distracted, or spiritually drained. We must set aside time for prayer, worship, and seeking God without compromise. If we don't, our spiritual hunger will be filled with things that do not satisfy: busyness, entertainment, and worldly distractions.

It's easy to let spiritual disciplines slip when life gets busy. Skipping prayer one day turns into two, then a week, and suddenly, we feel distant from God and wonder why we're struggling. But just like physical hunger, spiritual hunger must be fed regularly. When we don't nourish our spirits with God's presence, we start feeling heavy, overwhelmed, and confused.

We must be intentional about protecting our time with God. Setting a boundary around our spiritual life means prioritizing it above everything else: before work, before social media, and before anything that competes for our attention. Jesus set this example. Even in the midst of His demanding ministry, He often withdrew to be alone with the Father (Luke 5:16). If Jesus needed that time, how much more do we?

Spiritual boundaries also mean guarding who we allow to speak into our lives. Not everyone is meant to pour into us. If we surround ourselves with people who drain our faith, distract us from our purpose, or lead us into compromise, we need to reassess those relationships. The enemy often uses subtle influences to pull us away from God, so we must be discerning about where we invest our time and energy.

The Power of Saying No

Jesus Himself demonstrated boundaries. He withdrew to pray, said no to distractions, and rebuked anything that opposed His mission. Likewise, we must learn to say no. No to unhealthy habits, toxic relationships, and anything that draws us away from the abundant life God desires for us.

Saying no is one of the most powerful things we can do because every yes we give to something unhealthy is a no to something better. When we say no to processed junk food, we say yes to a healthier body. When we say no to negative self-talk, we say yes to confidence in Christ. When we say no to toxic influences, we say yes to peace.

The enemy wants us to live without boundaries because he knows it will keep us exhausted, distracted, and ineffective. But when we establish boundaries, we take back control of our health, mind, and spiritual life. We live with intention, clarity, and strength.

Boundaries Bring Freedom

Establishing boundaries is not about living in restriction but in freedom. It is about honoring the temple God has given us so we can live in clarity, strength, and purpose. When we set boundaries in our bodies, minds, and spirits, we create space for God to move. We experience peace, healing, and transformation.

A temple without walls is open to anything, good or bad. But a temple with strong walls and guarded gates can thrive, flourish, and fulfill its purpose. The same is true for us. When we build and maintain God-honoring boundaries, we walk in the fullness of His plan for our lives.

Strength for the Temple

Conditioning the Body, Mind & Spirit

When God calls us to step out in faith and act courageously in His name, we must trust in His promises of provision and protection. He does not call us to something and then abandon us; He equips us with the strength to carry it out. But strength is not something that happens overnight. Just like physical endurance is built through training and consistency, spiritual and mental resilience are developed through discipline, perseverance, and trust in God.

Strength Requires Preparation

Many people pray for strength in the moment of crisis, but true strength is cultivated before the battle begins. Jael, a woman known for her decisive action in Judges 4, demonstrated this. She had both the physical ability and mental resolve to act when the time came. Had she not been conditioned, physically strong enough to carry out the task and mentally prepared to step into a moment of divine purpose, she might have hesitated or failed.

The same applies to us. If we are weak in body, mind, or spirit, we may find ourselves unprepared for the moments when God calls us to take action. Strength does not come from waiting until we are faced with a challenge; it comes from consistent preparation.

- Physical Strength: If our bodies are not healthy, we will not have the endurance to carry out the work God has for us. When we are fatigued, weighed down, or sluggish from poor nutrition and neglect, we struggle to stand firm. Our temple must be conditioned through movement, proper nutrition, and rest so that when the time comes, we are ready to act.
- Mental Strength: Our minds must be trained to focus, discern, and push through resistance. If we do not develop mental discipline, we will cave under pressure, doubt ourselves, or allow fear to keep us from obedience. Renewing our minds daily in God's truth builds mental fortitude.
- Spiritual Strength: The foundation of all strength comes from the Spirit of God within us. If we are spiritually weak, disconnected from prayer, distant from His Word, and inconsistent in our faith, we will lack the confidence and clarity to step into our assignments with boldness.

Strength is Not Just for Us; It's for the Mission.

Jael's strength was not just for her own benefit; it was for God's greater purpose. In the same way, the strength we cultivate is not just for us to feel good or look good; it is for God's mission through us. Whether we are called to lead, serve, protect, or intercede, we must be equipped for the task.

If we are careless with our bodies, we may not have the stamina for the long road ahead. If we are careless with our minds, we may allow doubt or fear to talk us out of our calling. If we are careless with our spirit, we may become distracted, discouraged, or deceived.

Strength Must Be Maintained

Just as physical conditioning must be maintained through regular movement and nourishment, spiritual and mental strength requires ongoing effort. We cannot rely on yesterday's prayers, last month's disciplines, or a season of past breakthroughs to sustain us today.

- Stay in the Word: The Bible is our source of truth, wisdom, and endurance. If we are not continually consuming it, we will become spiritually malnourished.
- Practice Self-Control: The ability to say no to what weakens us and yes to what strengthens us is key to maintaining endurance. This applies to food, entertainment, relationships, and even our own thoughts.
- Build Resilience: Strength is tested in resistance. Instead of running from challenges, we should see them as opportunities for God to refine us. Growth happens when we push past discomfort and press into God's power.

God's Strength is Our Foundation

At the core of all, this is the truth that our strength comes from God. While we do our part in conditioning our temple, it is ultimately His power that sustains us. Psalm 18:32 says, *"It is God who arms me with strength and keeps my way secure."* When we align our bodies, minds, and spirits with Him, we become vessels that can be used mightily for His kingdom.

Strength is not just about being ready for the battle. It is about being prepared for the purpose. When the moment comes, will you be ready?

Encouragement for Single Moms: A Life of Example and Discipline

As a single mom, you face unique challenges, but let me encourage you: it can be done. You are not alone in this. God has equipped you with everything you need to not only survive but thrive. When you make the decision to reset your body, mind, and spirit in alignment with God's purpose, you are setting a powerful example for your children. You are teaching them about discipline, perseverance, and the importance of taking care of the body God has entrusted to you.

Remember, your children are watching. They see your strength in the way you handle your responsibilities, the way you make choices, and the way you prioritize your health. By choosing to honor God with your body, you're showing them the value of living with intention. You are building a legacy of health, faith, and strength that will impact them far beyond the years you are raising them.

It is beneficial to your children when you prioritize your health, not just for your well-being, but to demonstrate how to honor God in every area of life. As you choose to discipline your body and mind, you teach them that discipline isn't punishment, it's empowerment. Every step you take toward physical and emotional health is a step toward becoming the woman of God you were always meant to be. It is an example they will carry with them for the rest of their lives.

In this journey, remember that God sees your efforts. He knows the long nights, the worries, and the sacrifices you make. He sees your heart to do better, and He will meet you in those moments, strengthening you. Trust that as you reset, you're doing more than changing your body; you're building the foundation for the next generation. Your children will remember how you showed up, how you relied on God, and how you overcame obstacles with grace.

Do Not Worry About Food

Trusting God as Our Provider

One of the most well-known passages in the Bible about food and worry is found in Matthew 6:25-26:

"Therefore I tell you, do not worry about your life, what you will eat or drink; or about your body, what you will wear. Is not life more than food, and the body more than clothes? Look at the birds of the air; they do not sow or reap or store away in barns, and yet your heavenly Father feeds them. Are you not much more valuable than they?"

This verse is a powerful reminder that food is not meant to be our focus, nor something that causes us stress or obsession. If God provides for the birds, how much more will He provide for us? But in our modern world, food has become a source of worry in different ways. Some worry about having enough, while others obsess over calories, diets, and body image. Some use food to fill emotional voids, while others let it control them entirely.

Yet, God's Word calls us to trust Him rather than be consumed with thoughts about food.

The Spiritual Aspect of Food

Food was designed to nourish our bodies, but it was never meant to rule us. When we constantly worry about what to eat, how much to eat, or whether we will ever gain control over our cravings, we are essentially placing food in a position of power over us. This is not God's design.

Instead, Scripture reminds us:

- Man does not live by bread alone: *"Man shall not live on bread alone, but on every word that comes from the mouth of God."* (Matthew 4:4)
- God will satisfy us: *"For he satisfies the thirsty and fills the hungry with good things."* (Psalm 107:9)
- The kingdom of God is not about food : *"For the kingdom of God is not a matter of eating and drinking, but of righteousness, peace, and joy in the Holy Spirit."* (Romans 14:17)

When we reset our mindset, we recognize that food is a tool, not a master. It is meant to fuel us for the work God has called us to do, not to be an idol that we bow to in stress, cravings, or emotional struggles.

Breaking Free from Food Anxiety

Instead of fearing food or worrying about it, God calls us to seek Him first:

"But seek first his kingdom and his righteousness, and all these things will be given to you as well." (Matthew 6:33)

This means that when we prioritize God, when we focus on feeding our spirit first, He takes care of everything else, including our physical needs. When we are walking in alignment with Him, our relationship with food becomes healthy, disciplined, and peaceful.

Practical Steps for Resetting Your Mindset on Food

1. Pray Before You Eat: Not just as a habit, but truly thanking God for what He has provided and asking Him to help you steward it well.
2. Shift Your Focus: Instead of thinking of food as a reward, a comfort, or a burden, see it as fuel for God's work in your life.
3. Let the Word Be Your Bread: When cravings hit, turn to Scripture and prayer instead of immediately reacting to your desires.
4. Trust God's Provision: If He cares for the birds, He will care for you. Whether you struggle with overindulgence, restriction, or food-related anxiety, He is able to bring balance and freedom.

The moment we stop worrying about food and start trusting God with our bodies, we step into a place of peace, discipline, and true fulfillment.

The example of Jesus overcoming food temptation can serve as a powerful reminder that our bodies are not meant to be ruled by our immediate cravings. In the wilderness, when Jesus was tempted by the devil to turn stones into bread after 40 days of fasting, He responded with a profound truth: *"Man shall not live by bread alone, but by every word that comes from the mouth of God,"* (Matthew 4:4). Jesus, though physically weak and hungry, chose to rely on the strength of God's Word rather than give in to the pull of His flesh.

This moment reveals the deeper truth that the body is not our master, and what we feed it should align with God's purpose for our lives. Just as Jesus resisted the temptation to satisfy His immediate hunger, we too can resist our own cravings, whether for food or other comforts, by grounding ourselves in God's Word and His greater plan for us.

In this way, discipline is not a punishment but a way to honor God with our bodies and hearts. When we resist temptation and discipline ourselves, we are not only aligning our actions with God's purpose, but we also allow ourselves to hear His voice more clearly. Just like Jesus, who overcame the temptation to eat out of His physical need, we can overcome our cravings and find strength in the Word of God, creating space for spiritual clarity and growth.

When You Feel Like Giving Up

Victory is Coming

I get it. The weight of disappointment, exhaustion, and frustration can feel unbearable. You've tried, you've fought, and yet, here you are, wondering if it's even worth it anymore. But before you throw in the towel, let me remind you of something: You are not alone, and this is not the end of your story.

The enemy wants you to believe that nothing will ever change, that you'll always feel this way, and that giving up is your only option. But those are lies. The truth is, you were created with a purpose, and God's plan for you is greater than what you can see right now.

The breakthrough you've been waiting for might be just around the corner. The healing you need, the restoration you long for, and the peace you crave are not out of reach. Sometimes, the hardest battles come right before the greatest victories.

Isaiah 41:10 says, *"Fear not, for I am with you; be not dismayed, for I am your God; I will strengthen you, I will help you, I will uphold you with my righteous right hand."*

That's His promise to you. Strength when you're weak. Help when you're weary. A firm grip when you feel like you're slipping.

So breathe. Pause. Cry if you need to, but don't quit. Keep moving forward, even if it's just one small step at a time. The God who carried you this far isn't about to let you go now.

Hold on. Victory is coming.

Change the Way You Think and Speak to Yourself

The way you think and talk to yourself shapes your entire life. What you dwell on in your mind becomes what you believe in your heart, and what you believe in your heart determines how you live. If you constantly tell yourself, "I'll never change. I'm too far gone. I always fail," then that's the direction your life will take.

But here's the truth: You are not what the enemy says about you. You are not even what you feel about yourself on your worst days. You are who God says you are. And His Word is unshakable.

The enemy's greatest weapon is deception. He whispers lies, hoping you'll come into agreement with them. But you don't have to accept them. You have the power to take every thought captive and replace it with the truth of God's Word.

Recognizing the Lies and Replacing Them with Truth

- Lie: "I'm not good enough."
- Truth: "I am God's workmanship, created for good works." (Ephesians 2:10)
- Lie: "I always mess things up."
- Truth: "The Lord is my strength and my song; He has become my salvation." (Exodus 15:2)
- Lie: "No one cares about me."
- Truth: "I am loved with an everlasting love." (Jeremiah 31:3)
- Lie: "I will always struggle."

- Truth: "I am more than a conqueror through Christ." (Romans 8:37)
- Lie: "Nothing ever changes for me."
- Truth: "God is making a way in the wilderness and streams in the wasteland." (Isaiah 43:19)

Speak Life, Even When You Don't Feel It

At first, it might feel unnatural to speak the truth when you're used to negativity. But faith isn't about feelings; it's about standing on God's promises no matter what. Even when circumstances don't look different yet, your words and thoughts have the power to shift the atmosphere.

Start declaring:

- "I am strong in the Lord."
- "God's plans for me are good."
- "I am walking in healing and freedom."
- "The Spirit of God lives in me."
- "I am not a victim; I am victorious in Christ."

This isn't just self-help; this is spiritual warfare. Every time you replace a lie with the truth, you are tearing down strongholds. Every time you speak God's Word over yourself, you are aligning your mind with heaven.

Romans 12:2 says, *"Do not be conformed to this world, but be transformed by the renewing of your mind."* This isn't a one-time decision. It's a daily, intentional choice to reset your thoughts and reset your words.

And when you do? Your life will begin to change. Not because of your own strength, but because you are standing on the unshakable foundation of God's truth.

It's time for a reset. Speak life. Think the truth. Live free.

Speaking Life Over Your Temple

Instead of agreeing with sickness, exhaustion, and brokenness, begin declaring:

- "There is health, healing, and wellness in my house, which is the temple of the Holy Spirit."
- "My body is strong, healed, and whole in Jesus' name."
- "The same Spirit that raised Christ from the dead lives in me and brings life to my body." (Romans 8:11)
- "I walk in divine health, peace, and restoration."

The enemy would love for you to believe that sickness, stress, or poor health are just things you have to live with. But Jesus didn't die and rise again for you to live in a constant state of defeat. He came so that you would have life and have it abundantly (John 10:10).

The Temptation to Quit

The Battle for True Transformation

Why do we want to quit when we are so close to hitting our goal? The struggle to keep going when we're so close to our goal can be particularly intense because, at that moment, the pressure feels almost unbearable. It's like standing at the edge of a breakthrough but feeling paralyzed by the fear of what comes next. The temptation to settle arises when we feel overwhelmed, when the process of growth begins to unearth old wounds, insecurities, and patterns we've clung to for comfort. These habits, even though they're unhealthy, are familiar.

Change is uncomfortable, and often the closer we get to what we truly want, the louder the lies in our minds become. We tell ourselves that it's too much, or that we're not worthy, or that it's easier to stay where we are than to face the unknown.

It's important to understand that this feeling of wanting to quit isn't a reflection of our true potential, but rather a reflection of the emotional, spiritual, and physical battle that comes with transformation. Sometimes, we get so focused on the obstacles in front of us that we lose sight of the purpose behind it all. The reset process isn't just about changing our bodies, but about aligning ourselves with God's purpose. The mind and spirit are deeply intertwined with the physical, and as we work to reset one part, the others follow. When we hit that point of wanting to settle, it's often because we're in the thick of inner transformation.

At that moment, God invites us to press in deeper, to trust Him with the outcome, and to lean into the discomfort, knowing that He has already equipped us for what lies ahead. There's beauty in the breaking. There's strength in the stretching. Every step we take through the pain and the fear brings us closer to the true version of ourselves that God has designed. The reset is a spiritual process, an act of surrender, of leaning into His power and purpose rather than relying on our own strength.

Sometimes, we want to settle because we're afraid of success. Success means change, and change often brings new responsibilities, new expectations, and the weight of living up to our full potential. It's easier to stay in our current state, where we know what to expect, even if that state isn't where we're meant to be. But God doesn't call us to settle for mediocrity. He calls us to something greater, something that reflects His glory.

When we feel like quitting, it's vital to remind ourselves why we started. Reconnect with the vision and the purpose behind the reset. This isn't just about personal success; it's about honoring God with our bodies, minds, and spirits, and allowing His presence to transform us from the inside out. By pressing through the moments when we feel like giving up, we align ourselves more fully with His plan for our lives. And in that journey, we experience true freedom.

When you're focusing on a meal plan but others want to meet and it involves food, it's important to approach the situation with grace, wisdom, and balance. Here are some responses that honor God:

1. Gracious Acceptance: "I'd love to meet, but I'm currently focused on a specific meal plan for health reasons. How about we meet somewhere where I can stick to my plan, or perhaps we could focus on just the fellowship and conversation instead?"
2. Offer Alternatives: "I appreciate the invitation! Would it be okay if we meet at a place that has healthy options, or we could even bring our own meals and enjoy each other's company in a more relaxed setting?"
3. Transparency with Boundaries: "I'm in a season where I'm intentionally focusing on my health and meal plan to honor God with my body. I'd love to still connect, and perhaps we could do something that doesn't center around food?"
4. Express Intentions: "It's important for me to stay aligned with my goals right now. How about we spend time together in a way that doesn't focus on food, like a walk, or just sitting together for some quality conversation?"
5. Focus on Fellowship: "I'm in a season of focusing on my health, but I truly value our time together. How about we meet for coffee or tea, or take a walk instead? I'd love to spend time with you and not have food be the focus."
6. Invite Understanding: "I'm working on some personal health goals right now, and sticking to a meal plan is part of that. I'd still love to catch up, perhaps we can meet for a quick chat or a fun activity that doesn't involve food?"
7. Be Honest and Kind: "I've been feeling called to prioritize my health right now, so I'm sticking to a meal plan. But I'd

love to spend time with you, can we meet somewhere that doesn't tempt me off track, or maybe just meet for a coffee?"
8. Extend Love in Other Ways: "I really want to honor God with my choices, and that means I'm focusing on eating a certain way right now. That said, I'd love to see you, let's plan something fun that isn't centered on food."
9. Affirm the Importance of Relationships: "I'm so grateful for our friendship and would love to meet, but right now I'm focusing on sticking to a meal plan. How about we do something that isn't food-related, like going to a movie or just catching up over a walk?"
10. Redirect the Focus: "I'm in a season of focusing on my health and sticking to my meal plan, but that doesn't mean I don't want to connect! Let's plan something where we can just enjoy each other's company, like going for a hike or having a fun conversation."
11. Gentle but Firm Boundary: "Thank you for thinking of me! Right now, I'm in a place where I'm sticking to a specific eating plan to take care of my body. I'd love to get together at a time that doesn't revolve around food, though!"
12. Keep It Positive: "I'm in a season where I'm focusing on taking care of my health, so I'm sticking to a meal plan. But I'd love to meet up! Let's get creative and find something fun to do together that aligns with my current goals."

These responses honor both your meal plan and the relationships you're nurturing, showing that you value people over food while still staying committed to your goals.

When you respond with grace, honesty, and respect for your own boundaries, it not only shows that you are committed to your health and honoring God with your choices, but it can also create an opportunity for the other person to reflect on their own habits and choices. Here's how your responses may influence them:

1. Modeling Self-Discipline: When you share that you're prioritizing your health and meal plan, you're modeling self-discipline and intentionality. This can inspire others to think about their own health choices and how they might also benefit from being more mindful of what they consume.
2. Showing That Health Can Be a Priority: Your response emphasizes that taking care of your body and aligning your habits with your values is important. This can prompt the other person to consider how they might also be able to prioritize their own health in a balanced and God-honoring way.
3. Inviting Reflection on Priorities: By suggesting alternatives to food-centered activities (like walking, coffee, or other social options), you subtly invite the other person to reconsider what truly matters in their relationships. It shows that connecting with others doesn't need to revolve around food, which could spark a shift in how they approach socializing and spending time together.
4. Creating Space for Open Conversations: When you explain that you're focusing on your health as part of honoring God, you open the door for a deeper conversation about values and priorities. This could prompt the other person

to reflect on their own relationship with food, health, and their spiritual walk.
5. Encouraging Accountability: Your response can encourage the other person to think about how their own choices align with their goals or values. It may even encourage them to join you in making healthier decisions, fostering mutual support.
6. Inviting Positive Change Without Judgment: Your response avoids being critical or judgmental. It simply states your boundary and the reasoning behind it, which can lead the other person to reflect on their habits without feeling attacked. This can plant the seed for positive change in a way that feels empowering, not coercive.

Ultimately, when you live out your values and express them with kindness, you invite others to consider their own choices without making them feel pressured or judged. Your response can be a quiet but powerful invitation for them to consider making changes in their life, too.

1. Food as a Gift from God

God provides food for our nourishment and enjoyment:

- Genesis 1:29: "Then God said, 'I give you every seed-bearing plant on the face of the whole earth and every tree that has fruit with seed in it. They will be yours for food.'"
- Psalm 104:14-15: "He makes grass grow for the cattle, and plants for people to cultivate, bringing forth food from the earth: wine that gladdens human hearts, oil to

make their faces shine, and bread that sustains their hearts."

2. Eating in a Way That Honors God

- 1 Corinthians 10:31: "So whether you eat or drink or whatever you do, do it all for the glory of God."
- Romans 14:17: "For the kingdom of God is not a matter of eating and drinking, but of righteousness, peace, and joy in the Holy Spirit."

3. Self-Control and Moderation

- Proverbs 25:16: "If you find honey, eat just enough, too much of it, and you will vomit." (This speaks to moderation and not overindulging.)
- Philippians 3:19: "Their destiny is destruction, their god is their stomach, and their glory is in their shame. Their mind is set on earthly things." (A warning against making food an idol.)

4. Avoiding Legalism About Food

- The Bible warns against making food a source of division or unnecessary religious rules:
- Colossians 2:16: "Therefore do not let anyone judge you by what you eat or drink, or with regard to a religious festival, a New Moon celebration, or a Sabbath day."
- 1 Timothy 4:3-4: "They forbid people to marry and order them to abstain from certain foods, which God created to be received with thanksgiving by those who believe and who know the truth. For everything God

created is good, and nothing is to be rejected if it is received with thanksgiving."

5. Spiritual Food Is Even More Important

- While physical food is necessary, Jesus emphasized that spiritual nourishment is the highest priority:
- Matthew 4:4: "Jesus answered, 'It is written: Man shall not live on bread alone, but on every word that comes from the mouth of God.'"
- John 6:35: "Then Jesus declared, 'I am the bread of life. Whoever comes to me will never go hungry, and whoever believes in me will never be thirsty.'"

6. Caring for the Body as God's Temple

- 1 Corinthians 6:19-20: "Do you not know that your bodies are temples of the Holy Spirit, who is in you, whom you have received from God? You are not your own; you were bought at a price. Therefore honor God with your bodies."

This applies to how we nourish our bodies, exercise self-control, and treat food as part of our stewardship of God's gift. Food in the Bible is seen as both a blessing and a responsibility. It is meant to be enjoyed with gratitude, used in moderation, and never to become an idol. The ultimate focus should always be on honoring God, not just through what we eat, but in how we live.

A Healthy Vessel

The Essential to Carry Out His Purpose

A healthy, functioning body, your temple, is essential for living out God's purpose in your life. Your body is not just a physical structure; it is the vessel through which you fulfill God's will. When your body is healthy and working as designed, it becomes an instrument that enables you to serve others, glorify God, and carry out the work He has set before you.

God created your body with purpose. Psalm 139:14 says, *"I praise you because I am fearfully and wonderfully made; your works are wonderful, I know that full well."* Each part of you, from your heart to your muscles, was intentionally designed by the Creator. When your body is functioning as it was designed to, you experience the fullness of the life He intended for you.

A healthy body provides the energy, strength, and clarity you need to walk out your calling. When we neglect our physical well-being, we often experience fatigue, illness, and a lack of vitality that can hinder our ability to serve others or carry out the work God has called us to. In 1 Corinthians 9:27, Paul says, *"I strike a blow to my body and make it my slave so that after I have preached to others, I myself will not be disqualified for the prize."* He understood the importance of maintaining physical health to live out his spiritual mission effectively. A working temple equips you to fulfill your purpose without being hindered by physical limitations.

Furthermore, taking care of your body is an act of worship. Romans 12:1 urges us to offer our bodies as "a living sacrifice, holy and pleasing to God." Your physical well-being is directly tied to your spiritual health. When you honor your body, you honor God. Caring for it through proper nutrition, exercise, rest, and self-care shows gratitude for the life He's given you. It's about seeing your body not as an obstacle to your spiritual life, but as a vital partner in it.

A healthy body also gives you the mental and emotional stability needed to live with peace and joy. 3 John 1:2 says, *"Dear friend, I pray that you may enjoy good health and that all may go well with you, even as your soul is getting along well."* Health isn't just physical; it's holistic. When your body is healthy, your mind and spirit are better equipped to experience peace, clarity, and purpose. Emotional and mental well-being are deeply interconnected with physical health. When you take care of your temple, it affects your mood, energy levels, and overall sense of well-being.

Ultimately, a well-functioning temple reflects God's glory. Your body is a living testimony of God's creative power. It is a means through which you can experience His provision, strength, and grace. When you live in a way that honors your body, through mindful eating, movement, rest, and self-care, you reflect God's image in the best way possible. Your temple becomes a place where His Spirit can dwell freely, helping you live out the life He's called you to with passion, purpose, and vitality.

By embracing this truth, you recognize that your health is not just for your own benefit; it's for God's glory. When your temple is healthy and working as designed, you can be more effective in all areas of your life: spiritually, emotionally, and physically, bringing greater honor to God and fulfilling His purposes for you.

It's Not Hurting Anyone When I Overeat… Or Is It?

I used to believe that my eating habits were my business alone. If I wanted to eat beyond what my body needed, what was the harm? No one else was affected. But the truth is, everything we do, especially when it comes to our bodies, minds, and spirits, has a ripple effect.

Overeating wasn't just about food. It was about the moments when I felt unseen, unheard, or overwhelmed. It was a way to comfort myself, to create a false sense of control in a world that often felt chaotic. The problem? It didn't work. Instead of feeling comforted, I felt sluggish. Instead of feeling in control, I felt trapped in a cycle of regret and shame. And instead of feeling free, I felt bound.

The Bible tells us that our bodies are temples of the Holy Spirit (1 Corinthians 6:19-20). That doesn't mean God expects perfection, but it does mean He cares about how we treat the bodies He gave us. When I overate, I wasn't just hurting my health, I was dulling my spiritual sensitivity. I wasn't hearing God as clearly, I wasn't moving in the fullness of my calling, and I wasn't showing up as the best version of myself for my family, my ministry, or even the people God put in my path to love and serve.

But here's the beautiful thing about God, He doesn't just point out areas that need healing; He offers the healing. I had to come to Him, surrendering not just my eating habits but the pain, the stress, and the deep-rooted beliefs that made me think food was my answer.

Temple Reset isn't about following another diet or shaming yourself into change. It's about breaking free from the patterns that keep us stuck: physically, mentally, and spiritually. It's about allowing God to reset us so we can live with more energy, clarity, and purpose.

So, is it really not hurting anyone? I challenge you to ask yourself:

- Is my body functioning at its best so I can fully serve God and others?
- Am I using food to fill a spiritual, emotional, or mental void?
- Is my mind clear and my spirit free, or do I feel weighed down and distant from God?

The good news is, no matter where you are, there is always a reset available. God's grace is here. The question is, are you ready to step into it?

Healing is Your Portion

He is Faithful to Restore

Whether you need healing in your body, clarity in your mind, or renewal in your spirit, God is faithful to restore. Psalm 103:2-3 says, "Bless the Lord, O my soul, and forget not all His benefits, who forgives all your iniquities, who heals all your diseases."

No matter what has been spoken over your health, whether by doctors, family, or even your own thoughts, God has the final say. Declare His Word over your temple, align yourself with His truth, and walk in the wellness that is already yours in Him.

You are a temple. A house of healing. A dwelling place for God's presence. Walk in that truth.

Breaking Free from False Comforts

I was once weighed down by migraines, worry, and fear. These physical and emotional burdens felt like chains that kept me in a constant state of unrest. My body, hurting and exhausted, would crave comfort, but not from the source I truly needed, God. Instead, I turned to food as a false comfort, hoping it would provide temporary relief. But every bite only deepened the emptiness, and the cycle continued: the migraines persisted, the worry grew heavier, and I felt further away from the peace I desperately longed for.

It took time to realize that I was looking for comfort in the wrong places. What I needed wasn't something external to fill the void; it was a deep, spiritual reset. The kind of reset that could only come through surrendering my burdens to God, trusting in His healing power, and learning to find true peace in His presence.

I had to remind myself to never forget where I came from. The painful journey, the struggles with fear and anxiety, the false comforts I sought; they were part of my story, but they didn't define me. God had delivered me from so many things, and He had the power to rescue me from this, too.

God's Word became my refuge, and His truth began to heal not only my body but also my mind and spirit. He taught me that my body is a temple, worthy of His care, and that I didn't have to carry the weight of my struggles alone. Through prayer, faith, and a commitment to resetting my body, mind, and spirit in alignment with God's purpose, I was set free from the cycle of false comfort.

God's power to rescue isn't limited to a past rescue; it is ongoing. He's always ready to deliver us from the cycles that weigh us down if we let Him. Today, I walk in that freedom, knowing that true comfort comes from the Lord, and that He will always be my source of peace.

Clarity Through Purity

As I began to reset my body and mind, I realized something profound: when you aren't consumed with so much garbage food, you can hear God more clearly. The constant cravings, the unhealthy habits, and the endless cycle of indulgence clouded my mind and spirit. They were distractions that drowned out God's still, small voice.

When I started to focus on nourishing my body with what was truly good and aligned with His purpose, I found that my thoughts were clearer, my emotions more stable, and my connection with God deeper. I could hear His guidance more clearly, and His peace filled the spaces where the noise once resided.

It's amazing how when we honor our bodies with the right choices, the clutter of this world falls away. Our ability to discern God's voice increases because we are no longer numbed by the things we've used to fill the void. In the quiet, we can hear the whisper of His love, direction, and healing.

Living a Life of Dedication: Holding On in the Darkest Times

Living a life of dedication isn't always easy. It's not just about the good days when everything feels aligned, but also about remaining steadfast in the face of hardship. There have been times in my own journey when my health was at stake, and the physical pain was so intense that it felt like I was spiraling into a dark, spiritual place. The pain overwhelmed me, and the fear of what might come next was consuming.

In those moments, it felt like everything was slipping through my fingers. But even in the darkness, I held onto God's word. I didn't always feel strong, and sometimes it was hard to see how anything could change. But His word was my anchor. I chose to believe His promises, every word spoken over my life, and I saw

Him move in miraculous ways, healing me in ways that I could not have imagined.

God's word has a power that transcends our circumstances. It speaks life into places that feel dead; it brings light to the darkest moments, and it heals in ways that doctors, treatments, and even time cannot. As I clung to His promises, I experienced His healing, not only in my body but also in my spirit. I began to see how He had been working all along, even in the midst of my pain, shaping me, strengthening me, and leading me toward deeper trust in Him.

There will be times in life when we face trials that seem insurmountable. But when you choose to dedicate every area of your life to God, your body, your mind, your spirit, you are inviting Him to show up, to lead you, and to bring you through the storm. Even when it feels like there's no way out, God is always present, always working behind the scenes, and always faithful to His word. Trusting in Him, holding onto His promises, and living a life of dedication means that you don't have to walk through the darkness alone. He will show up, and He will bring healing in miraculous and unexpected ways.

The Importance of Discipline and Killing the Flesh

One of the hardest battles I faced was fighting cravings and my tendency to eat to numb the pain I was feeling. It was a constant struggle, but I quickly realized that every time I gave in to those cravings, 20 minutes later I would feel worse than before. In those moments, I had to fight back, not with willpower alone, but by reminding myself of what the Bible says and the end goal God has set before me.

In those difficult times, I often had to turn to God's Word for strength. The Scriptures are clear about the importance of discipline in all aspects of our lives, especially in caring for our bodies. I began to understand that my health wasn't just about feeling good or looking good; it was about being able to do what God had called me to do. Health is wealth, and if I'm not healthy, I can't fulfill my purpose in this life.

Each time I resisted the urge to give in to unhealthy habits, I was not just choosing physical well-being but spiritual strength. The more I disciplined my body, the clearer I could hear God's voice. I started seeing that taking care of myself wasn't just a personal endeavor; it was an act of obedience.

This is the power of killing the flesh. It's not about denying ourselves for the sake of self-punishment, but about saying no to the temporary pleasures of this world so we can live in full alignment with God's calling. It is not punishment; it is purpose. And when we discipline our flesh, we become stronger spiritually, emotionally, and physically, enabling us to live out our purpose with clarity and strength.

Healing the nervous system from trauma starts with understanding that your body holds onto the memories of past pain. When we experience trauma, the nervous system gets stuck in a state of fight, flight, or freeze. Healing begins when we prioritize rest, safety, and self-regulation. Practicing deep breathing, meditation, and prayer helps to reset the nervous system, signaling to your body that it's safe to release the tension. Physical movement, such as gentle stretches, yoga, and exercise, also plays a vital role in releasing trapped emotions and calming the nervous system. By nurturing your body with healthy food and making space for emotional and spiritual healing, you can rebuild resilience, allowing your body to feel safe, grounded, and connected to the present moment. This healing process is crucial for aligning your body, mind, and spirit with God's purpose for your life.

To practice healing your nervous system, start by creating a safe, peaceful environment where you can slow down and reconnect with yourself. This can involve setting aside quiet time for prayer, journaling, or deep breathing exercises. A simple practice like 4-7-8 breathing (inhale for 4 seconds, hold for 7, exhale for 8) can help shift your body out of stress and back into calm.

Next, start to move forward by taking small steps toward safety and connection. Begin by listening to your body and honoring what it needs. If you're feeling triggered or anxious, give yourself permission to pause, breathe, and ask God for guidance. Movement is another way to move forward; whether it's stretching or even a walk in nature, these actions help to release the stored trauma in your body.

It's also important to build a support system, seek counseling, engage in group therapy, or reach out to trusted friends and mentors who can walk alongside you in the healing process. As you rebuild your sense of safety and trust in God, you'll be able to move forward, not from a place of fear or survival, but with strength, peace, and purpose.

Remember, healing is not linear. It's okay to take breaks, be gentle with yourself, and seek God's presence in every step. Trust that, as you move forward, your nervous system will gradually rewire itself to a place of peace, allowing you to live in the fullness of what God has for you.

I want to address the way social media bombards us with food content, endless videos of people eating massive portions, indulging in extreme cravings, or glorifying unhealthy foods. These videos aren't just harmless entertainment; they play a role in feeding unhealthy habits, normalizing overeating, and keeping people trapped in cycles of cravings, emotional eating, and even addiction to food.

Social media algorithms push what keeps people watching, and food is one of the biggest triggers. Whether it's mukbangs, fast food hauls, or "What I Eat in a Day" videos that showcase excessive or unrealistic portions, these posts don't encourage discipline or mindful eating. Instead, they fuel the flesh, pushing people to overindulge, making food the focus of comfort and entertainment rather than nourishment.

For someone trying to reset their temple, body, mind, and spirit, these videos can be a stumbling block. They keep food at the forefront of our minds, reinforcing cravings and making it harder to hear from God clearly. If we are constantly consuming content that glorifies indulgence, it becomes much harder to practice self-control and honor our bodies the way God intended.

I've learned that what we consume, both physically and mentally, shapes our habits. If we feed our minds with content that promotes excess, our actions will follow. That's why part of the reset process is being intentional about what we allow into our eyes and ears. Discipline isn't about deprivation; it's about freedom, freedom from unhealthy cycles, from feeling enslaved to cravings, and from anything that dulls our ability to hear God's voice.

A true reset means stepping away from what feeds the flesh and stepping into what strengthens the spirit. It's about replacing mindless scrolling with mindful choices, letting go of what doesn't serve us, and allowing God to truly nourish us in every way.

The Power of Fasting

Realigning Our Hearts with Him

Fasting is a powerful discipline that resets not only the body but also the mind and spirit. It's a way to break unhealthy attachments to food, realign our hearts with God, and deepen our reliance on Him rather than on physical sustenance.

Fasting: A Key to Resetting the Temple

1. Spiritual Realignment: Fasting shifts our focus from physical cravings to spiritual nourishment, reminding us that *"man shall not live by bread alone, but by every word that proceeds from the mouth of God"* (Matthew 4:4). It's a way to silence distractions and seek God with greater clarity.
2. Breaking Food Strongholds: If food has become an idol, a comfort, or an obsession, fasting helps break its control. It teaches us that our bodies don't rule us; God does.
3. Detoxing Body & Spirit: Physically, fasting gives the digestive system a rest, promoting healing and renewal. Spiritually, it helps cleanse the heart, allowing God to reveal areas where we need healing or deliverance.
4. Restoring Self-Control: Fasting strengthens discipline, reminding us that we don't have to give in to every craving. This carries over into other areas of life, helping us develop self-control and a deeper dependence on the Holy Spirit.

5. Strengthening Prayer & Intimacy with God: Fasting and prayer go hand in hand. Scripture shows that breakthroughs often come when fasting is combined with prayer (Daniel, Esther, Jesus in the wilderness). It's a way to humble ourselves and invite God's power into our struggles.

A true reset involves not just what we eat but also when we step away from food to seek God. Whether through intermittent fasting, extended fasting, or a fast from specific foods, the goal is always the same: resetting the body, mind, and spirit to function in alignment with God's purpose.

We were created to worship God, not food or anything else that takes His place in our hearts. When food becomes an obsession, whether through overeating, emotional eating, or an excessive focus on diets and body image, it can become an idol, something we turn to for comfort, satisfaction, or control instead of God.

The Bible warns against this kind of misplaced worship. Philippians 3:19 says:

"Their end is destruction, their god is their belly, and they glory in their shame, with minds set on earthly things."

This verse reminds us that when we let our appetites rule us, we drift away from God's purpose. Instead of allowing food to control us, we should surrender our desires to God and seek Him first.

Jesus also set an example when He said in Matthew 4:4:

"Man shall not live by bread alone, but by every word that proceeds from the mouth of God."

This verse shows that true sustenance comes from God's Word, not just physical food. Our bodies are temples of the Holy Spirit (1 Corinthians 6:19-20), and when we reset our focus on worshiping God instead of being controlled by food, we align ourselves with His perfect design for our lives.

Fasting

Gaining Clarity & Breaking Strongholds

Fasting, turning down your plate, is one of the most powerful ways to reset your body, mind, and spirit. It's not just about food; it's about surrender. When you deny your flesh, you create space for God to move. You gain clarity, break strongholds, and align yourself with His will.

So many of us run to food for comfort, for control, or out of habit, but fasting breaks those cycles. It forces you to confront what truly fills you, because if food is your source, you'll always be hungry for something more. But when God is your source, you'll be sustained in ways food never could.

Fasting played a major role in my transformation, revealing areas of my life that needed healing and correction. When I turned down my plate, God turned things around.

Fasting changed my life in ways I never expected. It wasn't just about food; it was about resetting my body, mind, and spirit to be in alignment with God's purpose. When I fasted, I could hear from God more clearly. The noise that usually cluttered my mind faded away, and His voice became unmistakable. Distractions or sluggishness no longer clouded my thoughts. Instead, I felt sharp, focused, and spiritually in tune.

Physically, I had more energy. I wasn't weighed down or exhausted like before. My body felt lighter, and I wasn't constantly battling fatigue. It was as if my system had been given a reset, and I could move through my days with a renewed sense of strength.

But what impacted me most was the excitement I felt to spend time with God. Fasting wasn't a burden; it was an invitation. I wasn't just going through the motions of prayer; I was encountering Him in a fresh and powerful way. It reignited my passion for His presence and deepened my hunger for more of Him.

Fasting wasn't just about what I was giving up; it was about what I was gaining. And what I gained was far greater than anything I could have imagined.

Here's the truth: food was never meant to control us; we were meant to have dominion over it. But sugar and processed carbs have a way of keeping people in bondage, not just physically, but mentally and spiritually. They create cravings, spikes and crashes, brain fog, and even emotional instability. When your body is constantly inflamed, your mind and spirit suffer too.

Cutting out sugar and refined carbs isn't just about weight loss; it's about breaking free from the cycle of addiction and stepping into a life of clarity, strength, and discipline. When I made this shift, I realized how much food had been a distraction, numbing emotions I didn't want to face. But once I committed to clean eating, I saw how it sharpened my focus, improved my energy, and deepened my connection with God.

The Bible speaks of the body as a temple, and just like a physical temple, what we bring into it matters. Clean eating is a form of stewardship; it's about honoring the body God gave you so you can walk in the fullness of His purpose. When you strip away the things that weigh you down, you open yourself up to greater strength, endurance, and spiritual breakthroughs.

This journey isn't about deprivation; it's about transformation. It's about fueling your body with real, life-giving foods so that you can function at your best: mentally, physically, and spiritually. When you remove the things that slow you down, you position yourself for the reset that God wants to bring into your life.

A Sweet-Smelling Aroma to God

Offering Living Sacrifices

Throughout Scripture, we are called to honor God with our bodies, minds, and spirits, as they are temples of the Holy Spirit (1 Corinthians 6:19-20). But what does it mean to honor God with our temples, and how does it become a sweet-smelling aroma to Him? To understand this, we must consider the concept of offerings and sacrifices in the Bible.

In the Old Testament, God instructed His people to bring offerings, whether they were animals, grains, or incense, into His presence. These offerings, when made with a pure heart and in obedience to God's commands, were seen as a fragrant offering, a sweet-smelling aroma to the Lord (Leviticus 1:9, Ephesians 5:2). The aroma signified that the sacrifice was pleasing to God, an act of worship that was wholehearted and aligned with His will.

This principle applies to us today. When we embark on a Temple Reset, we are, in essence, offering ourselves to God as living sacrifices (Romans 12:1). As we realign our lives with His purpose and choose to care for our bodies, renew our minds, and strengthen our spirits, we are offering a fragrant sacrifice.

But what makes this reset a "sweet-smelling aroma" to God? It is not the mere act of discipline, but the heart behind it. God does not delight in empty rituals or outward actions; He delights in a contrite heart and a desire to please Him (Psalm 51:17). When we reset our temple, we are choosing to prioritize His will over our own desires, to lay aside distractions, and to surrender every part of our being to Him. This heart of surrender, of obedience, is what makes our lives a sweet fragrance before God.

Furthermore, a sweet-smelling aroma speaks to God's desire for purity. Just as incense was used to symbolize prayers rising before the Lord, the way we care for our bodies and minds symbolizes our prayers and our relationship with Him. When we cleanse our hearts of unhealthy thoughts, habits, and attitudes, and when we nourish our bodies with food that glorifies God, we allow the sweet fragrance of holiness to rise up to Him. We remove the clutter and the chaos, and in its place, we create an environment where God's presence can dwell richly.

Doing a Temple Reset means we are actively making choices that reflect God's character in us. It means we are allowing Him to shape us, to mold us, and to renew us so that we can walk in the fullness of His purpose for our lives. Every time we choose to say no to self-sabotage, every time we decide to nourish our bodies with healthy food instead of giving in to cravings that harm us, we are participating in an act of worship. These small acts of obedience accumulate, creating a life that is fragrant to the Lord.

The process of resetting is not only about physical health, but spiritual renewal as well. As we grow in discipline and strength, we also grow in intimacy with God. Our minds are clearer, our hearts are more sensitive to His voice, and our actions reflect His goodness. Both the spiritual and physical combined create a life that is pleasing to Him, a life that rises like incense before the throne of God.

This transformation is not only about removing what is unhealthy but also about filling our lives with what is good, true, and beautiful. By resetting our temple, we are making space for God's presence to dwell more fully within us. The choices we make to honor our bodies and minds are acts of worship that please God, and these choices create a life that reflects His glory. Our lives become a living testimony of His power to transform, and this transformation is what pleases Him the most.

Many people hesitate to fully trust Jesus with their lives because they fear He will limit them. They worry that following Him means giving up freedom, that He will impose rigid rules and restrictions that make life smaller and less enjoyable. But the reality is quite the opposite.

When Christ enters your life, He doesn't confine you; He liberates you. Instead of making life dull and religious, He makes it vibrant and full of purpose. He doesn't diminish who you are; He awakens who you were always meant to be. Rather than narrowing your world, He expands it, opening your eyes to things you never noticed before and giving you a depth of understanding, joy, and fulfillment that nothing else can offer.

You may be living a good life right now, but God wants to give you a better life, not one weighed down by empty pleasures, fleeting highs, or the pressures of striving to measure up, but one that is truly abundant. A life where you are fully alive, deeply loved, and completely free.

This same truth applies to how we care for our bodies, our temples. Many people resist making changes to their health because they fear it will mean losing out on enjoyment. They think eating clean, being disciplined, and taking care of their bodies will feel restrictive, just another set of rules that make life smaller. But just like trusting Jesus, surrendering this area of your life actually leads to more freedom, not less.

When you stop filling your body with processed, unhealthy foods that weigh you down, you begin to experience the energy, clarity, and strength God intended for you. You're not just existing; you're thriving. Your mind becomes sharper, your emotions more stable, and your spirit more in tune with God's presence. Suddenly, you can hear Him more clearly, move through life with greater purpose, and step into the fullness of who He created you to be.

God doesn't call us to take care of our bodies to punish us or deprive us; He calls us to it so we can truly live. He wants us to be free from the addictions, cravings, and unhealthy cycles that keep us bound. He wants to remove the things that are dulling our senses and keeping us from fully experiencing His presence.

When you see health through this lens, it's no longer about restriction; it's about expansion. It's about stepping into a life that is more abundant, more fulfilling, and more aligned with God's purpose. What may seem like sacrifice at first is actually a divine exchange, trading what is lesser for what is greater. And just like with our faith, when we trust God with our health, we realize He isn't trying to take away our joy; He's trying to give us more of it.

Prayers & Declarations

How to Use These Prayers & Declarations

Meal Prayers: Inviting God into Every Bite Prayer Before Eating: A Heart of Gratitude

Pray Before & After Meals: Use these prayers to invite God into your eating habits.

1. Speak Declarations Daily: Declare these truths over yourself every morning, before meals, or whenever you face temptation.
2. Write Down Key Declarations: Keep them in a journal, on your phone, or on sticky notes as reminders.
3. Personalize Them: Modify the declarations to speak directly to your personal struggles and victories.

Father, thank You for this meal. I receive it as a gift from Your hands, meant to nourish my body and sustain my strength. Help me eat with gratitude, wisdom, and self-control. Let my choices bring glory to You. In Jesus' name, Amen.

Prayer for Self-Control & Discernment

Lord, I ask for wisdom in my eating today. Help me to stop when I am satisfied and not be driven by cravings or emotions. I choose to eat with intention, not indulgence. Fill me with Your Spirit, and let my hunger be first and foremost for You. Amen.

Prayer When Facing Temptation

God, I feel tempted to eat in a way that does not honor my body or You. Give me the strength to say no when necessary and the wisdom to know what my body truly needs. I take my thoughts captive and choose to be led by Your Spirit, not my flesh. Thank You for empowering me to make wise choices. Amen.

Prayer After Eating: A Heart of Contentment

Lord, thank You for providing this food and for satisfying me. I trust that You know what my body needs, and I submit my appetite to You. May this meal fuel me to do the work You have set before me today. I praise You for being my true source of satisfaction. In Jesus' name, Amen.

Daily Declarations: Speaking Life Over Your Health

Speak these daily declarations over yourself to renew your mind and reinforce biblical truths about food, health, and freedom.

Declarations for a Healthy Relationship with Food:

- "Food is a gift, not a god. I receive it with gratitude, not obsession."
- "I eat to fuel my body, not to feed my emotions."
- "I am satisfied in Christ, not in food."
- "I have self-control because the Holy Spirit lives in me."
- "I honor my body as God's temple by making wise food choices."

Eating to fuel your body rather than to feed your emotions is crucial for both physical and mental well-being. When you eat for fuel, you're providing your body with the nutrients it needs to function optimally, giving you energy, mental clarity, and overall health. However, when eating is driven by emotions such as stress, sadness, or boredom, it can lead to unhealthy habits, weight fluctuations, and a cycle of guilt and dissatisfaction.

Why It Matters:

Physical Health: Food is meant to nourish and sustain you, supporting your metabolism, immune system, and organ function. Emotional eating often leads to consuming unhealthy, processed foods that can cause inflammation, fatigue, and other health issues.

Mental & Emotional Well-being: Emotional eating may bring temporary relief, but it doesn't address the root of the emotions. Instead, it can create a cycle where food becomes a coping mechanism rather than a source of nourishment.

Spiritual & Mind-Body Connection: When food becomes an idol or an escape, it can distance you from relying on God for emotional and spiritual strength. Learning to see food as a gift to steward rather than a crutch helps align your body with God's purpose.

Shifting Your Perspective:

Recognize emotional triggers and seek God first instead of turning to food for comfort.

Choose nutrient-dense foods that give life and energy rather than foods that leave you sluggish and depleted.

Develop habits like prayer, movement, or journaling to process emotions in a healthy way.

When you eat to fuel your body, you regain control over your health and allow your emotions to be guided by truth rather than temporary cravings. It's a step toward freedom, discipline, and honoring the temple God has given you.

Declarations for Freedom from Food Idolatry:

- "Food does not control me; Christ has set me free!"
- "I am not a slave to cravings; I am led by the Spirit."
- "I do not find comfort in food; I find comfort in God alone."
- "I break all unhealthy attachments to food and step into God's perfect plan for my health."
- "God is my provider, and I trust Him to meet all my needs: physically, emotionally, and spiritually."

Declarations for Self-Control & Strength:

- "I have the mind of Christ, and I make choices that honor Him."
- "I am disciplined, strong, and in control of my body through the power of the Holy Spirit."
- "I listen to my body and eat in moderation, not in excess."
- "I do not let stress or emotions dictate my eating habits."
- "Every meal I eat is an opportunity to glorify God."

Declarations for Confidence & Identity in Christ:

- "My worth is not determined by my weight, size, or what I eat. It is found in Christ alone."
- "I am beautifully and wonderfully made by God."
- "I am growing in wisdom, strength, and self-discipline every day."

- "God's grace is sufficient for me, even when I struggle."
- "I trust God's process for my body and my health."

Living a disciplined life according to the Bible involves aligning your actions with God's will and developing habits that reflect His guidance. Here are some key steps based on Scripture:

"Beloved, I wish above all things that thou mayest prosper and be in health, even as thy soul prospereth." 3 John 1:2.

1. God Cares About Every Part of You

   - This verse shows that God is not just concerned with our spiritual well-being but also our physical health and prosperity.
   - True prosperity isn't just financial; it's about having a healthy soul, mind, body, and life.

2. Spiritual Growth is the Foundation

   - The phrase "even as thy soul prospereth" means that our outward blessings should align with our inner spiritual health.
   - A prosperous soul means a close relationship with God, peace, joy, and spiritual maturity.

3. Health and Prosperity Flow from a Healthy Soul

   - When our soul is right with God, it impacts our mental, emotional, and even physical well-being.
   - This verse reminds us to seek first God's kingdom (Matthew 6:33), knowing that when our soul prospers, everything else follows.

Application to Life

- Prioritize your spiritual health through prayer, the Word, and obedience.
- Take care of your physical health because your body is a temple (1 Corinthians 6:19-20).
- Trust God for provision and blessings, knowing He wants you to thrive.

When food becomes an idol, it takes a place in our lives that should belong to God. Idolatry isn't just about worshiping statues; it's anything we rely on more than God for comfort, security, or fulfillment. Here's how making food an idol can be harmful:

1. It Replaces Dependence on God

    - Instead of turning to God for peace, joy, or healing, we turn to food for comfort or escape (emotional eating).
    - Jesus said, "Man shall not live by bread alone, but by every word that proceedeth out of the mouth of God." (Matthew 4:4). Food sustains the body, but only God can satisfy the soul.

2. It Can Lead to Unhealthy Habits

    - Overeating, binge eating, or obsessing over food can lead to physical health issues (weight gain, disease, fatigue).
    - It can also create a cycle of guilt and shame, especially if we feel out of control.

3. It Distracts from God's Purpose

    - If food controls our thoughts, cravings, and decisions, it steals our focus from what God is calling us to do.

- Paul reminds us, "All things are lawful for me, but I will not be brought under the power of any." (1 Corinthians 6:12).

4. It Can Be a Form of Bondage
   - Food is a good gift from God, but when it masters us, it becomes a form of slavery.
   - Jesus came to set us free, including from unhealthy attachments (Galatians 5:1).

5. Breaking Free from Food Idolatry
   - Recognize it: Be honest if food has taken an unhealthy place in your life.
   - Turn to God for satisfaction: Replace emotional eating with prayer, worship, and Scripture.
   - Practice self-control: "The fruit of the Spirit is self-control." (Galatians 5:22-23).
   - Honor your body: Eat to fuel, not to numb or escape.

Breaking free from food idolatry is a process of surrendering control to God, renewing your mind, and developing healthy habits. Here's a biblical and practical approach to overcoming it:

1. Recognize & Repent
   - Be honest with God: Confess if food has taken an unhealthy place in your life.
   - Repentance means change: It's not just feeling bad; it's deciding to walk in a new direction with God's help.
   - Pray for deliverance: Ask the Holy Spirit to break any stronghold of emotional eating, obsession, or dependence.

2. Renew Your Mind (Romans 12:2)
   - Replace food as comfort with God's Word: Meditate on Scriptures about God's provision and satisfaction.
   - Declare truth: Say things like, "God is my provider, not food," or "My body is a temple, and I will treat it with care."
   - Ask the right questions: Before eating, ask:
   - Am I actually hungry?
   - Is this fueling my body or feeding an emotion?
   - Have I prayed about how I feel?
   - Practice Self-Control (Galatians 5:22-23)
   - Set healthy boundaries: Avoid situations that lead to binge eating (e.g., stress, boredom, certain triggers).
   - Plan meals intentionally: Eat for fuel, not feelings.
   - Fast & pray: Fasting teaches discipline and resets your dependence on God, not food.
3. Find Freedom in God, Not Guilt
   - Grace over guilt: If you slip up, don't condemn yourself. Confess, realign, and keep moving forward.
   - Celebrate progress: Every time you turn to God instead of food, you're winning the battle.
   - Seek accountability: A trusted friend, mentor, or support group can help.
   - Shift Your Focus to Kingdom Purpose
   - Instead of thinking about food all the time, focus on:
   - Spending time in God's presence.
   - Serving others.
   - Pursuing your calling with energy and strength.

Key Scriptures to Meditate On

- Matthew 4:4: Man shall not live by bread alone, but by every word of God.
- 1 Corinthians 10:31: Whether you eat or drink, do all to the glory of God.
- Philippians 4:13: I can do all things through Christ who strengthens me.

If your body matched your spiritual health, how strong would you be?

Nourish your spirit like you do your body, through prayer, the Word, and God's presence.

Temple Reset

21-Day Scripture Reflection, Prayer & Journaling Guide

<u>Week 1</u>

Resetting the Mind

(Renewing Your Thoughts)

Day 1

Surrendering to God's Will

- Scripture: Romans 12:2- "Do not conform to the pattern of this world, but be transformed by the renewing of your mind."
- Reflection: Today marks the beginning of a journey. Let's reflect on how we have been shaped by the world's standards: expectations, values, and pressures. Surrendering to God's will requires us to break free from those molds and allow Him to renew our thinking. This is a process of transformation, and it begins in the mind. How can we make space for God to reshape the way we think and live?

_____

_____

_____

_____

_____

_____

_____

_____

_____

Day 2

Overcoming Fear & Anxiety

- Scripture: 2 Timothy 1:7 : "For God gave us a spirit not of fear but of power and love and self-control."

- Reflection: Fear often holds us back from stepping into God's best for us. Today, let's confront the fears that may have been controlling us. Fear is not from God, it's a tool used by the enemy to keep us from walking in power, love, and self-control. What would your life look like if you fully embraced the boldness God has given you?

_____

_____

_____

_____

_____

_____

_____

_____

_____

Day 3

Fixing Your Eyes on Jesus

- Scripture: Hebrews 12:2: "Fixing our eyes on Jesus, the pioneer and perfecter of faith."
- Reflection: We live in a world full of distractions that pull our focus away from what really matters. Jesus is the perfect example of how to live a life in alignment with God's purpose. Today, reflect on what has been stealing your focus and how you can return your eyes to Jesus. What does it look like to make Him the center of your thoughts and actions?

_____

_____

_____

_____

_____

_____

_____

_____

_____

Day 4

Every Thought Captive

- Scripture: 2 Corinthians 10:5: "We demolish arguments and every pretension that sets itself up against the knowledge of God, and we take captive every thought to make it obedient to Christ."

- Reflection: Our thoughts are powerful. They shape our emotions, actions, and ultimately, our lives. As we take every thought captive, we choose to reject negative, self-destructive thoughts and replace them with the truth of God's Word. What are some lies you've believed, and how can you replace them with the truth of who God says you are?

_____

_____

_____

_____

_____

_____

_____

_____

Day 5

Gratitude Reset

- Scripture: 1 Thessalonians 5:16-18: "Rejoice always, pray continually, give thanks in all circumstances; for this is God's will for you in Christ Jesus."

- Reflection: Gratitude is an attitude that shifts our focus from lack to abundance. Today, take time to reflect on the blessings in your life, no matter how small. Cultivating a thankful heart can transform your perspective and draw you closer to God. What are you most thankful for today, and how can you carry that gratitude with you throughout the day?

_____

_____

_____

_____

_____

_____

_____

_____

_____

Day 6

Speaking Over Yourself

- Scripture: Proverbs 18:21: "The tongue has the power of life and death, and those who love it will eat its fruit."
- Reflection: The words we speak are powerful. They shape not only how others see us but also how we see ourselves. Today, reflect on the words you've spoken over your life. Are they words of life and encouragement, or do they reflect doubt and negativity? Speak life today by declaring God's promises over your life.

_____

_____

_____

_____

_____

_____

_____

_____

_____

Day 7

The Power of Resting in God

- Scripture: Matthew 11:28-30: "Come to me, all you who are weary and burdened, and I will give you rest."

- Reflection: Rest is a vital part of our spiritual, mental, and physical well-being. We are called to take our burdens to God and find rest in His presence. Reflect on your current pace of life. Are you allowing yourself?

_____

_____

_____

_____

_____

_____

_____

_____

_____

_____

Week 2

Resting the Body

Discipline

&

Health as Worship

Day 8

Your Body is God's Temple

- Scripture: 1 Corinthians 6:19-20: "Do you not know that your bodies are temples of the Holy Spirit, who is in you, whom you have received from God?"

- Reflection: Your body is a sacred vessel, created by God and meant to honor Him. Reflect on how you treat your body; does it reflect respect and honor for God? What changes can you make to care for your body in a way that reflects your love and gratitude for Him?

_____

_____

_____

_____

_____

_____

_____

_____

_____

Day 9

Eating With Intention

- Scripture: 1 Corinthians 10:31: "So whether you eat or drink or whatever you do, do it all for the glory of God."
- Reflection: Eating is not just a physical need; it is an opportunity to honor God. Reflect on the foods you choose and how they impact your body. Are you eating with intention, or do habits and emotions dictate your food choices? How can you honor God through the meals you eat today?

Day 10

Killing the Flesh, Strengthening the Spirit

- Scripture: Galatians 5:16-17: "So I say, walk by the Spirit, and you will not gratify the desires of the flesh."
- Reflection: The desires of the flesh are often in direct opposition to the desires of the Spirit. Reflect on the areas where your flesh has been in control, whether it's food, unhealthy habits, or other distractions. Surrender these areas to God today, asking for strength to live according to His will and not your flesh.

Day 11

Self-Control is a Gift

- Scripture: Galatians 5:22-23: "But the fruit of the Spirit is love, joy, peace, forbearance, kindness, goodness, faithfulness, gentleness and self-control."

- Reflection: Self-control is not a form of punishment, but a fruit of the Spirit that empowers us to live in alignment with God's will. Reflect on where you may be lacking in self-control and ask God to help you grow in this area. How can you strengthen your spirit to resist temptation and stay disciplined in your choices?

_____

_____

_____

_____

_____

_____

_____

_____

_____

Day 12

Your Body Needs Rest

- Scripture: Psalm 127:2: "In vain you rise early and stay up late, toiling for food to eat, for he grants sleep to those he loves."
- Reflection: Rest is a gift from God, not a luxury. Reflect on how you balance work and rest. Are you honoring God by giving yourself the rest you need? What can you do today to prioritize rest and trust in God's provision?

Day 13

Moving Your Body for God's Glory

- Scripture: Colossians 3:23: "Whatever you do, work at it with all your heart, as working for the Lord, not for human masters."

- Reflection: Exercise is a way to honor God with our bodies. Reflect on the physical activity you engage in and how you can view it as an act of worship. Whether it's walking, dancing, or lifting weights, do it with gratitude and dedication to the Lord.

_____

_____

_____

_____

_____

_____

_____

_____

_____

Day 14

Breaking Free From Bondage to Sin

- Scripture: Philippians 3:19: "Their mind is set on earthly things."
- Reflection: Food is meant to nourish our bodies, not control us. Reflect on whether you have allowed food to become an emotional crutch or idol. What steps can you take to break free from the hold that food has over you? How can you turn to God instead of food when you feel the urge to comfort yourself?

_____

_____

_____

_____

_____

_____

_____

_____

Week 3

Resetting the Spirit

Spiritual Renewal

&

Purpose

Day 15

God is Your Source of Strength

- Scripture: Isaiah 40:31: "But those who hope in the Lord will renew their strength."

- Reflection: We often look to our own strength to carry us through difficult times, but God is our true source of strength. Reflect on areas where you've been relying on your own abilities instead of trusting in God's strength. Where do you need His strength today?

Day 16

Walking in Discipline, Not Punishment

- Scripture: Hebrews 12:11: "No discipline seems pleasant at the time, but painful. Later on, however, it produces a harvest of righteousness and peace."

- Reflection: Discipline is not punishment; it's a tool used by God to shape us. Reflect on how you view discipline in your life. How can you see it as an opportunity for growth and spiritual maturity? In what areas do you need more discipline?

Day 17

Self-Sabotage & Breaking Free

- Scripture: Romans 7:15: "I do not understand what I do. For what I want to do I do not do, but what I hate I do."

- Reflection: We all struggle with self-sabotage, doing things we know are not good for us. Reflect on patterns in your life where you've sabotaged your own progress. What steps can you take today to break free from this cycle?

Day 18

Hearing God More Clearly

- Scripture: John 10:27: "My sheep listen to my voice; I know them, and they follow me."
- Reflection: Hearing God's voice is essential for walking in His purpose. Reflect on the distractions that may be keeping you from hearing His voice clearly. How can you quiet your mind and spirit to listen for God's guidance today?

Day 19

Your Life as a Sweet-Smelling Aroma to God

- Scripture: 2 Corinthians 2:15: "For we are to God the pleasing aroma of Christ."

- Reflection: Our lives are meant to be an offering to God, a sweet-smelling aroma that pleases Him. Reflect on how your actions, thoughts, and decisions can be pleasing to God. What can you do today to live in a way that honors Him?

_____

_____

_____

_____

_____

_____

_____

_____

_____

_____

Day 20

Never Forget Where You Came From

- Scripture: Deuteronomy 8:2: "Remember how the Lord your God led you all the way in the wilderness these forty years."

- Reflection: It's important to never forget where we came from and what God has delivered us from. Reflect on the journey God has taken you on and how He has rescued and restored you. How can you share your testimony to encourage others?

_____

_____

_____

_____

_____

_____

_____

_____

_____

_____

_____

Day 21

Fully Surrendered & Walking in Purpose

- Scripture: Proverbs 3:5-6: "Trust in the Lord with all your heart and lean not on your own understanding."
- Reflection: The final step is fully surrendering to God and trusting Him to lead you in the purpose He has for your life. Reflect on how you can take one step today toward walking in that purpose. What does full surrender look like for you?

_____

_____

_____

_____

_____

_____

_____

_____

_____

_____

Conclusion

Temple Reset

As we come to the end of this journey through Temple Reset, I pray that you've experienced a transformation, not just in your physical body, but in your mind and spirit as well. Our bodies are sacred temples, entrusted to us by God. Throughout this book, we've explored how aligning our physical health with His will can open doors to deeper connection, greater clarity, and a more profound understanding of our purpose in Him.

Remember, Temple Reset is not a one-time event, but a continual process. It's about choosing every day to honor God with your body, to live with discipline and intentionality, and to recognize that true health isn't just about what we see on the outside, but what's happening on the inside. It's about your heart, your mind, and your relationship with God, all working in harmony.

And I want to remind you of this truth: You are not alone. In those moments when it feels hard or overwhelming, know that God is right there with you, walking alongside you every step of the way. He has not given you a spirit of fear, but of power, love, and a sound mind (2 Timothy 1:7). You have the strength, the wisdom, and the courage you need to take action and live in alignment with His purpose for your life. Trust that He has equipped you to make these changes, and that every decision you make, no matter how small, brings you one step closer to the life He's called you to live.

You can do this. There will be challenges, but with God's help, you will rise above them. Every time you choose discipline over temptation, health over convenience, and peace over chaos, you are honoring God with your temple. And He will give you the grace to keep moving forward, no matter how many times you stumble.

Now that you've been equipped with the tools and insights to reset your temple, I challenge you to take action. Don't wait for the perfect moment. Start today. Whether it's taking a step toward better health, making the choice to nourish your body with good food, or committing to a consistent movement routine, take that step in faith. Know that every small decision adds up to a life that reflects God's purpose and glory.

If you feel compelled, I invite you to join a community of like-minded individuals who are on the same journey of transformation. Share your story, your struggles, and your victories. You are not alone in this process. Together, we are stronger. There is power in community, in lifting each other up, and in encouraging one another to keep going when things get tough.

As you move forward, always keep this in mind: God has equipped you to live a life full of purpose, health, and vitality. Your body is a gift, a temple of His Holy Spirit, and by honoring it, you honor Him.

Call to Action

Start today. Reset your temple. Reset your life. If you've been moved by the messages in this book, I encourage you to share it with others. Let's spread the message of hope, discipline, and health to those who need it most. Join me on this journey of transformation, and together we will rise in strength, purpose, and faith.

Feel free to connect with me through social media or reach out via email at templereset@gmail.com to share your story or ask questions. You're not just resetting your temple; you're resetting your life in alignment with God's purpose. You can do this. Let's do it together!

About the Author

Joni Wilkinson

Joni Wilkinson is a speaker, teacher, and advocate dedicated to seeing people set free, healed, and delivered. As the Founder and Executive Director of One's Purpose, an anti-trafficking organization, Joni works to rescue and restore lives through education, outreach, and faith-based healing.

Her personal journey of overcoming trauma, breaking free from cycles of self-sabotage, and realigning her body, mind, and spirit with God's purpose has shaped her message. Temple Reset is born out of her firsthand experience of battling cravings, emotional eating, and misplaced discipline, learning that true health is not just physical but deeply spiritual. Through this book, she shares how surrendering to God's process brings clarity, strength, and transformation.

Beyond her advocacy work, Joni is also a tax strategist, mentor, and mother, passionate about equipping others to live in total freedom.

Resources: Connect with the Author

Thank you for joining me on this Temple Reset journey! If this book has impacted you or if you'd like to connect, I'd love to hear from you.

You can reach me through:

- Email: templereset@gmail.com
- Social Media: IG: @temple_reset

Your stories, questions, and testimonies mean so much to me. Let's continue growing together in body, mind, and spirit!

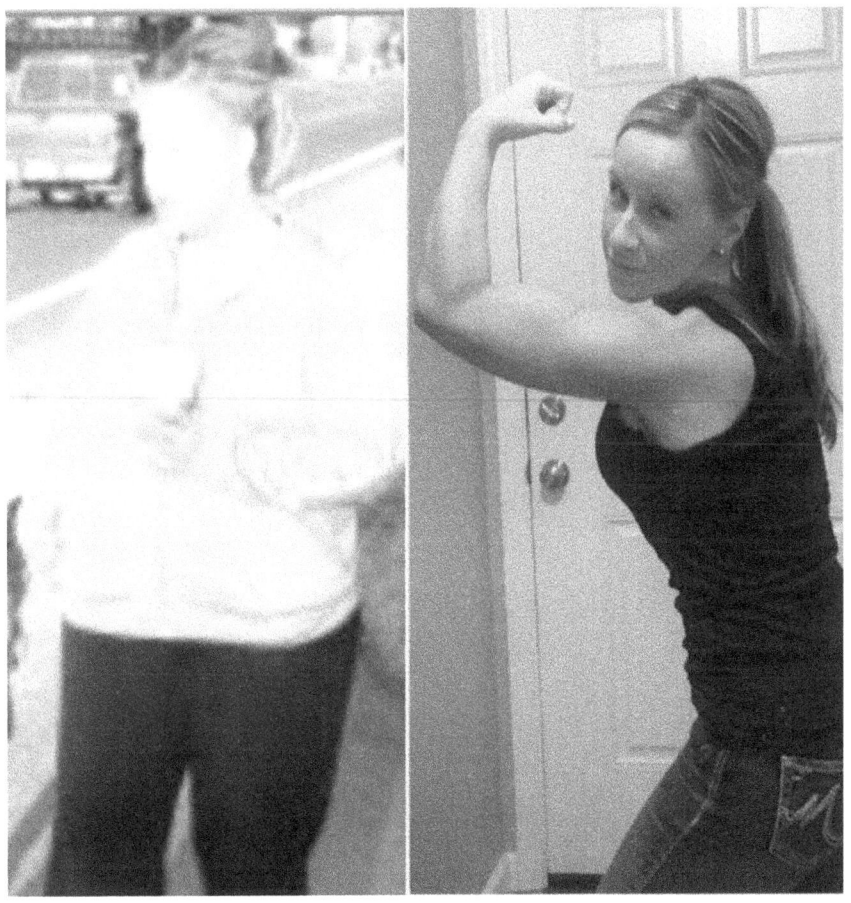

www.ingramcontent.com/pod-product-compliance
Lightning Source LLC
Chambersburg PA
CBHW052031030426

42337CB00027B/4953